Challenges in Program Evaluation of Health Interventions in Developing Countries

Barbara O. Wynn, Arindam Dutta, Martha I. Nelson

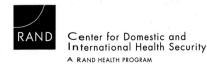

Center for Domestic and
International Health Security
A RAND HEALTH PROGRAM

This work was sponsored by the Global Health Policy Research Network, managed by the Center for Global Development, with funding from the Bill and Melinda Gates Foundation, under contract No. DHR-5-1-02. Partial funding was also provided by the Martin Foundation and by the RAND Corporation. This research was produced within RAND Health's Center for Domestic and International Health Security. RAND Health is a division of the RAND Corporation.

Library of Congress Cataloging-in-Publication Data

Wynn, Barbara O.
    Challenges in program evaluation of health interventions in developing countries / Barbara O. Wynn, Arindam Dutta, Martha I. Nelson
      p. ; cm.
    "MG-402."
    Includes bibliographical references.
    ISBN 0-8330-3852-4 (pbk. : alk. paper)
    1. World health. 2. Medical policy. I. Dutta, Arindam, 1976– II. Nelson, Martha I. III. Title.
    [DNLM: 1. Program Evaluation—methods. 2. World Health. 3. Communicable Disease Control—methods. 4. Developing Countries. 5. Health Policy. 6. Vaccination—methods. WA 530.1 W988c 2005]

RA441.W96 2005
362.1—dc22

                                  2005024410

The RAND Corporation is a nonprofit research organization providing objective analysis and effective solutions that address the challenges facing the public and private sectors around the world. RAND's publications do not necessarily reflect the opinions of its research clients and sponsors.

RAND® is a registered trademark.

A profile of RAND Health, abstracts of its publications, and ordering information can be found on the RAND Health home page at www.rand.org/health.

Published 2005 by the RAND Corporation
1776 Main Street, P.O. Box 2138, Santa Monica, CA 90407-2138
1200 South Hayes Street, Arlington, VA 22202-5050
201 North Craig Street, Suite 202, Pittsburgh, PA 15213-1516
RAND URL: http://www.rand.org/
To order RAND documents or to obtain additional information, contact
Distribution Services: Telephone: (310) 451-7002;
Fax: (310) 451-6915; Email: order@rand.org

Preface

This monograph provides an overview of issues related to program evaluation for health projects in developing countries. It is intended to promote the understanding that program evaluation is a critical component of any health intervention and to stimulate discussion on ways to raise the level of program evaluation and increase the resources and technical capacity needed to evaluate health interventions in developing countries. At the request of the sponsor of this study, this monograph focuses on issues surrounding evaluation of vaccination campaigns and interventions for HIV/AIDS, tuberculosis, and malaria. The intended audience for this report includes policymakers and organizations that fund health interventions in developing countries.

This work was sponsored by the Global Health Policy Research Network, managed by the Center for Global Development, with funding from the Bill and Melinda Gates Foundation, under contract No. DHR-5-1-02. Partial funding was also provided by the Martin Foundation and by RAND Corporation internal funds. This research was produced within RAND Health's Center for Domestic and International Health Security. RAND Health is a division of the RAND Corporation. A profile of the Center, abstracts of its publications, and ordering information can be found at www.rand.org/health/healthsecurity/.

Contents

Figures

Tables

Summary

A recent editorial in the *Journal of the American Medical Association* noted that the effectiveness of many health interventions in developing countries has not been proven. The editorial called for increased international support and collaboration to provide the infrastructure to evaluate global health interventions and move toward evidence-based global health (Buekens, 2004). Interventions that are effective in developed countries may not be effective in developing countries that have differing social, economic, cultural, and infrastructure factors that may affect how a project is implemented and the project's outcomes. Rigorous program evaluation of interventions in various resource-limited settings is needed to determine which interventions will work most effectively and to spend scarce resources wisely.

In a well-designed evaluative strategy, evaluation at each phase of a project informs the phases that follow and generally involves

- a formative evaluation during the project's developmental phase to clarify objectives and to refine the project design (including the evaluation strategy and data requirements), while taking into account the cultural environment and other local factors that influence how a project is implemented
- process evaluations throughout the project implementation phase to provide timely feedback on how the intervention has been implemented and what might be done to improve it operationally to achieve desired outcomes

- an impact evaluation to assess the net effects of the intervention and whether the intervention's goals were reached.

When supported by strong process evaluations, an impact evaluation provides information that can be used to design interventions in new sites that take advantage of the knowledge, experience, and "lessons learned" in similar cultural environments. To inform decisions on future program design, an evaluation model should provide for wide dissemination of findings from rigorous impact evaluation. Impact evaluations establish whether there is a causal chain of events (or "causal chain") between an intervention and observed outcomes. In order to attribute observed changes to an intervention, one must understand what changes would have occurred in the absence of the intervention, all else being equal. The challenge here is to control for any other factors that might explain the observed changes and to identify and measure the indirect effects of the intervention. Because one cannot directly measure what would have occurred without the intervention, a comparison must be made to a control group, or the program evaluation model must incorporate statistical controls. Statistical techniques that are commonly used to control for other factors include the following:

- Randomized control trials that compare at an intervention site those who were part of the intervention and those who were not
- Randomized cluster trials that compare populations at the intervention site with populations at a control site
- Quasi-experimental designs that use non-random means to construct experimental and control groups
- Pre- and post-regression comparisons.

Within the general model for program evaluation, various methodologies must be utilized selectively to develop and convey the information that is most pertinent to the goals and objectives of the particular project being evaluated. The challenge in this case is to develop an evaluative strategy that is most suitable to (1) the intervention's scope, design, and purpose; (2) its potential for being scaled up or replicated elsewhere; and (3) the potential value of the information that will be generated from the evaluation. This challenge is greatest when assessing heath outcomes and other impacts of health interventions in developing countries, for which the assumed benefits of many interventions remain unproven, and for which methodological issues, evaluative capacity, data limitations, and resource constraints make impact evaluations difficult to accomplish.

Despite the acknowledged benefits of randomized studies, the great majority of outcome evaluations continue to use standard regression-analysis methodologies. Some high-quality evaluations have demonstrated the value of rigorous impact assessments using randomized clinical trials or cluster analysis, but they are noteworthy exceptions. Our review of the literature and selected evaluations indicates that for the most part there is a considerable gap between "best practices" in program evaluation and the evaluative strategies actually being used.

Actions that might promote impact assessments of large-scale interventions fall into three broad interrelated categories: increasing support for impact evaluations, enhancing evaluative capacity, and improving evaluation methodologies.

Actions to Increase Support for Impact Evaluations

Developing Priorities for Impact Evaluation

A formal framework for deciding when an impact assessment would be appropriate could help funding agencies to think more systematically about their evaluative strategies. Typically, the size and complexity of an evaluation matches the size of a project and is proportional to the amount of resources invested in the project. However, evaluation should not be proportioned according to project size, but instead, more importantly, to the pre-existing amount of evidence that is predictive of the project's effect, the significance of the *disease burden* (the contribution of a disease to premature death and disability), and the policy relevance of the intervention. *Ex ante* evaluation designs are likely to be less time- and resource-intensive and more rigorous than post-implementation designs. Moreover, decisionmaking on an evaluation strategy during the formative evaluation stage may counteract some of the selection biases that are likely to occur with *ex post* selection of comparison groups and the bias against evaluating unsuccessful programs.

Building a Case for Impact Evaluation

The case for impact evaluation rests on two premises: (1) Knowing what works is important to wise investment of scarce resources for health projects and (2) knowing the impacts of successful, cost-effective interventions will generate additional investments in health. Funding organizations should think of impact evaluations as providing an "international public good" with benefits extending far beyond the benefits that accrue from decisions being made within individual organizations (Duflo, 2003). Case studies illustrating how impact evaluations have made a difference in funding priorities and program design are needed. These case studies should not only provide examples of where and how impact evaluations have led to decisions to scale up or replicate programs, but also where they have led to design modifications or to curtailing projects and reallocating funds to more effective interventions.

Encourage Multidisciplinary Evaluation Designs

Public health has shifted away from a purely medical approach to providing services toward a more fully integrated, multidimensional view of public health as being inextricably connected to larger social, behavioral, psychological, and economic factors. As public health programs collaborate with programs in other disciplines such as education and economic development, the evaluation methods typically used in the health, education, and economic fields also must undergo a type of integrative mixing. The strongest impact assessments harmoniously blend process evaluations and other non-quantitative assessments with quantitative analysis.

Funding Incentives

Funding organizations could create financial incentives, such as the following, to encourage more-rigorous impact evaluations.

- Conditional or staged funding could be used to encourage formative evaluations and prospective evaluation designs, so that the required data and evaluation metrics are established at the outset of the intervention.
- Most projects have specific funds intended for use in program monitoring and evaluation activities. An explicit dollar set-aside for an impact evaluation would safeguard funds for this purpose and assure that those funds are not diverted to ongoing monitoring activities.
- Grants for evaluation activities would be more attractive to government administrators than would loans for this purpose (Duflo, 2003).
- Matching grants, or outright grants, from international funding organizations could be a way to encourage both nongovernmental organizations and government programs to undertake evaluations.

Actions to Improve Evaluative Capacity

This section briefly discusses a number of steps that could be taken to increase the resources available for evaluation and the technical expertise of evaluators of health interventions in developing countries.

Facilitate Use of Evaluation Methodologies

Researchers are developing standards for reporting of methods, data, and outcomes to facilitate interpretation of program evaluations (Campbell et. al, 2004; Kirkwood, 2004). Funding organizations might consider establishing a "warehouse" for evaluations of health interventions and making this warehouse of information readily available to researchers via the Internet.

Increase Technical Capacity of Independent Evaluators

To build program evaluators' expertise, funding agencies should consider collaboratively sponsoring one or more independent multidisciplinary evaluation organizations. These organizations could

- serve as a resource for researchers on evaluation methodologies and issues
- conduct high-priority, randomized impact evaluations that could be used as "best practices" models for evaluation
- provide training and technical assistance for health-services research in developing countries
- maintain an easily accessible repository and/or gateway for evaluations of public-health interventions in developing countries and literature on evaluation methodologies and issues
- foster testing of new evaluation methodologies
- establish partnerships between local projects and researchers
- encourage further standardization of reporting of evaluation findings and of indicators.

Increase Local Evaluation Capacity

A delicate balance exists between involving local participants in an evaluation process and maintaining the rigor—such as standardized indicators, survey methods, and statistical techniques—needed for credible impact evaluations. Collaborative models that strive for this balance need to be developed and tested, so that evaluation activities can both build local evaluation capacity and contribute to evidence-based health interventions.

Disseminate Research Findings

Knowing what works and what does not work, with respect to both an entire project and individual components of the intervention, requires having results from both successful and unsuccessful projects being made available. This initiative requires not only stepping up the intensity of impact evaluation efforts but also widely disseminating the findings from those efforts.

Actions to Improve Evaluation Methodologies

Although statistical techniques to support impact evaluations have been developed, additional research in several areas would improve evaluations in terms of increasing the quality of the evaluations and making them less costly and time-consuming, which in turn would make them more attractive to funding organizations. Some areas that warrant additional consideration include the following:

- Conducting baseline and trend surveys during the program-design stage.
- Using a logical framework model to evaluate programs when randomized controlled trials are not possible.
- Developing rapid measurement techniques to secure the quick-snapshot data that are needed to gain at least a basic sense of trends and real-world program impact.
- Confirming that a strong link exists between the surrogate markers (proxy measures for a desired outcome measure that are used when directly measuring outcomes is not feasible) and the desired outcomes.
- Assessing the efficacy of evaluating "tracer" interventions, which reflect the key components of the entire intervention, to judge the overall true effectiveness of the entire program.
- Developing better indicators to measure contextual factors— such as organizational capacity and leadership commitment— which may affect the likelihood of an intervention's success and/or be indirectly affected by the intervention.
- Standardizing indicators to measure the nonbiological effects of health interventions on individuals, their families, and their communities.
- Strengthening ongoing data-collection systems and standardizing measures to reduce the costs of data collection for evaluations and to facilitate cross-site comparisons.

Increasing global support for program-impact evaluations, enhancing evaluative capacity, and improving evaluation methodologies should help to close the gap between "best practices" in program evaluation and evaluative strategies actually in use. There is general agreement among the public-health community that rigorous program evaluation of interventions in various resource-limited settings is needed to determine which interventions will work most effectively and to spend scarce resources wisely. What is not clear, however, is the extent to which incremental improvements in program-evaluation rigor produce information of sufficient strength to guide evidence-based, global-health policymaking.

Current evaluation levels clearly are insufficient. However, the scope of future evaluations must be carefully calibrated to match the significance of the intervention, and evaluation techniques must be carefully selected so that they achieve the desired level of precision in the information being sought. Researchers must be upfront about any limitations in the ability of their research methods to capture a range of effects, and they must explore new methods for capturing larger effects. This work may require greater amounts of qualitative reasoning, because the need for greater statistical rigor may exclude important broad insights. Indeed, as the evidence-based public-health movement presses for more-rigorous evaluation of intervention programs, the evaluations themselves must be continuously scrutinized for appropriateness.

Acknowledgments

We would like to thank the RAND staff who participated in a brainstorming session on program evaluation: John Adams, James Dewar, Richard Hillestad, Emmett Keeler, Yee-Wei Lim, Peter Mendel, James Quinlivan, Gery Ryan, Brian Stecher, and James Zazzali. Thomas Croghan provided insights that helped frame the issues discussed in this paper. We would also like to acknowledge the work done by Sara Bleich, a former RAND intern, who investigated the existing international data systems used to track HIV/AIDS.

We appreciate and benefited from the thoughtful comments of William Butz, Gery Ryan, Ruth Levine, and an anonymous reviewer. We appreciate the administrative assistance of Kathryn Khamsi in preparing an earlier version of this document.

Acronyms

ART	anti-retroviral treatments
BSS	Behavioral Surveillance Survey
CB-DOTS	Community-Based Directly Observed Therapy Short-Course
CDC	Centers for Disease Control and Prevention
CIOMS	Council for International Organization and Medical Sciences
CONSORT	Consolidated Standards of Reporting Trials
CPS	Contraceptive Prevalence Survey
DALY	disability-adjusted life years
DHS	Demographics and Health Survey
DOTS	Directly Observed Therapy Short-Course
FHI	Family Health International
HIV/AIDS	Human Immunodeficiency Virus/Acquired Immune Deficiency Syndrome
IFPRI	International Food Policy Research Institute
IPT	isoniazid prevention therapy
LQAS	lot quality assurance sampling
MDR	multi-drug resistant
MICS	Multiple Indicator Cluster Survey
NBER	National Bureau of Economic Research
OECD	Organization for Economic and Cooperative Development

PI	prevention indicator
PLWHA	people living with HIV/AIDS
PMTCT	preventing mother-to-child transmission
PRS	prevention research synthesis
QALY	quality-adjusted life years
RBM	roll back malaria
RCT	randomized control trial
RHS	Reproductive Health Survey
STI	sexually transmitted infections
TB	tuberculosis
TREND	Transparent Reporting of Evaluations with Nonrandomized Designs
UN	United Nations
UNAIDS	Joint United Nations Programme on HIV/AIDS
UNFPA	United Nations Populations Fund
UNICEF	United Nations Children's Fund
USAID	United States Agency for International Development
VCT	voluntary counseling and treatment
WFS	World Fertility Study
WHO	World Health Organization

CHAPTER ONE

Introduction

Purpose of the Study

A recent editorial in the *Journal of the American Medical Association* noted that the effectiveness of many health interventions in developing countries has not been proven. The editorial called for increased international support and collaboration to provide the infrastructure to evaluate global health interventions and move toward evidence-based global health (Buekens, 2004). Interventions that are effective in developed countries may not be effective in developing countries that have differing social, economic, cultural, and infrastructure factors that may affect how a project is implemented and the project's outcomes. Rigorous program evaluation of interventions in various resource-limited settings is needed to determine which interventions will work most effectively and to spend scarce resources wisely.

This report is intended to promote understanding of why evaluation is a critical component of any health intervention and to stimulate discussion on ways to increase the capacity to evaluate health projects and make evaluation of health interventions in developing countries more rigorous. We provide an introductory overview of various approaches, methodologies, and issues related to program evaluation for health projects in developing countries, and cite other sources of information on various evaluation techniques. We conclude by identifying research and other actions that could be taken by funding organizations that would facilitate impact evaluations of large-scale health interventions.

Program Evaluation in Developing Countries

Evaluation should be conducted throughout the various stages of an intervention, starting with the project design and ending with an assessment of ultimate outcomes. At any given stage of an intervention, the focus, scope, and technical issues will vary depending on the intended purpose of the evaluation at that stage. A well-designed evaluative strategy generally involves the following steps:

- a formative evaluation during the project's developmental phase to clarify objectives and to refine the project design (including the evaluation strategy and data requirements), while taking into account the cultural environment and other local factors that influence how a project is implemented
- process evaluations throughout the project implementation phase to provide timely feedback on how the intervention has been implemented and what might be done to improve it operationally to achieve desired outcomes
- an impact evaluation to assess the net effects of the intervention and whether the intervention's goals were reached.

Impact evaluations establish whether there is a causal chain of events (or "causal chain") between an intervention and observed outcomes. There may be a direct cause-and-effect linkage in the chain (e.g., vaccination for polio has a direct effect on an individual's immunity from polio) or the cause-and-effect linkage may be indirect (e.g., the impact of polio immunization campaigns on the national infrastructure for disease surveillance). The causal chain may involve a series of cause-and-effect linkages, some of which may be upstream (i.e., precede the intervention under evaluation), horizontal (i.e., cause-and-effect factors that involve individuals, such as family members, and organizations not directly participating in an intervention), or downstream (i.e., take place after an intervention, such as longer-term impacts on an individual or the community). To establish the causal chain and attribute observed changes to an intervention, it is important to understand what changes would have occurred in the absence of the intervention, all else being equal. The challenge in determining the effectiveness of an intervention is to control for any other factors that might explain the observed changes and to identify and measure the indirect effects of the intervention.

In the subsections below, we provide an overview of the public health issues on which we focus in this report—vaccination campaigns, Human Immunodeficiency Virus/Acquired Immune Deficiency Syndrome (HIV/AIDS), malaria, and tuberculosis—and the evaluation challenges they present. The interventions for each of these four public health areas have unique characteristics that pose their own set of challenges for impact evaluation.

Vaccination Campaigns

The World Health Organization (WHO) estimates that more than two million deaths in 2002 were from diseases for which vaccines are already available, and almost 1.5 million of those deaths were children (WHO, 2003b). A 2003 Global Immunization Score Card showed that only 26 percent of developing countries meet an 80 percent benchmark for routine immunization coverage, and a majority of developing countries has not yet introduced newly available vaccines, such as a vaccine for Hib (*Haemophilus influenzae* type b, which causes some forms of pneumonia and meningitis), which killed 413,000 children under the age of 5 in 2002. Over the past decade, immunization coverage of DTP3 has stagnated far below targets for sub-Saharan Africa and South Asia after rapid improvement in coverage throughout the 1980s, according to WHO/UNICEF estimates (Vaccine Assessment and Monitoring Team, 2004).

Because the efficacy of vaccinations is well established, and because vaccinations target diseases that occur early in childhood, evaluations of the effects of vaccines follow relatively short causal chains. Evaluators generally assume what the immunization effects of vaccination will be and rely on simple counts of vaccinated individuals to measure effectiveness; evaluators do not need to measure differences in disease prevalence.

However, persistent shortfalls in vaccine coverage have two implications for program evaluation. First, impact evaluations should consider not only whether the goals of an intervention were reached in terms of numbers of immunizations but also what accounted for the success or failure of a vaccination campaign. More information is needed on the broader determinants of the success of a vaccination campaign so that lessons learned and best practices can be considered when designing other vaccination campaigns. Second, more attention should be given to the downstream effects generated by immunization campaigns. The polio eradication initiative illustrates the indirect benefits of a health intervention. In addition to eradicating the disease from many areas, the polio program strengthened both immunization systems in general and the global health infrastructure, including worldwide networks of laboratories, surveillance systems, human resources, and vaccine-delivery equipment (Davey, 2002; Levine and What Works Working Group, 2004). Polio immunization campaigns also serve as platforms for providing basic health care services to children who had never before received medical attention. Currently, both polio and measles vaccination campaigns serve as channels for delivering vitamin A (Davey, 2002).

Broader impact evaluations that consider the indirect effects of vaccination campaigns could potentially demonstrate any additional benefits from those campaigns (and whether any trade-offs with routine immunizations and other preventive services are associated with vaccination campaigns) and lead to increased political support for them.

Malaria

Malaria causes more than 300 million acute illnesses and at least one million deaths annually, primarily among children in the tropical and subtropical regions of the world. Deteriorating health systems, increased resistance to drugs and insecticides, and environmental changes have led to an increase in malaria over the past two decades. Malaria poses intervention challenges as a vector-borne disease with no consistently effective vaccine and high resistance to treatment.

The public-health debate on malaria centers on the relative value of bed nets as an effective long-term strategy for malarial containment. To measure the effectiveness of this intervention, program evaluation must go beyond counts of distributed nets to substantiate a downstream causal pathway—i.e., the evaluation must also determine the degree to which people use bed nets appropriately and whether treating the nets with insecticide has a noticeable effect on the disease burden of the individuals using nets. Researchers might also try to determine if applying insecticides to bed nets lowers the population of mosquitoes in the environment or alters evolutionary pressure on viral character, which would confer indirect benefits on the community in which the intervention took place. The question of disease burden raises an issue regarding whether the unit of observation for gauging an intervention's effectiveness should be just the individuals who were provided with bed nets or the entire community in which the intervention takes place.

The long-term sustainability of the bed-nets intervention has been in question in part because some study findings have suggested that bed-net use in infancy might increase mortality in older children though delayed acquisition of immunity to malaria. Results from a two-year community randomized trial in Kenya, followed by continued surveillance of adherence and mortality rates for an additional four years, are encouraging in this regard. The researchers found sustained bed-net usage over the six-year study period and found no differences in the mortality rates in older children who had bed nets as infants and those who had not (Lindblade et al., 2004). The evaluation design for the Kenya study illustrates limitations that ethical considerations may pose for evaluation. For reasons of equity and community acceptance, insecticide-treated bed nets were distributed to control households at the end of the initial two-year trial, and bed nets were retreated with insecticide throughout the post-intervention surveillance period. Thus, the question of what happens to the mortality rates for children who are protected by bed nets in infancy after they are exposed to normally high malaria transmission remains unanswered.

Tuberculosis
WHO estimates that in 2002 eight million persons developed active tuberculosis (TB) and two million died from the disease, with 90 per-

cent of the active cases and deaths occurring in developing countries. The persistence of TB over the past decade has been primarily due to lack of government commitment to TB control, poorly managed TB-control programs, poverty, population growth, and a significant rise of TB cases in HIV-endemic areas (WHO, 2002a).

Directly Observed Therapy Short-Course (DOTS) is an internationally accepted cost-effective strategy to control TB that consists of five key elements:

- Government commitment to sustained TB control
- Detection of TB cases through sputum smear microscopy among people with TB symptoms
- Regular supply of high-quality anti-TB drugs
- Six to eight months of regularly supervised treatment
- Reporting systems to monitor treatment progress and program performance.

Globally, only 37 percent of the estimated number of TB patients received treatment under the DOTS strategy in 2002, with an 82 percent average success rate for treatment. As a broad-scale social intervention, the DOTS strategy does not lend itself to randomized controlled trials and poses evaluative challenges—for example, determining why TB rates in the former Soviet Republic have fallen in recent years and understanding the implications that these falling TB rates might have for TB-control programs in other countries (Dyer, 2005).

Multi-drug resistant (MDR) TB is far more costly to treat than TB strains that can be treated with standard short-course therapy. Cost-effective treatment regimens still need to be identified for MDR TB. Because interrupted or discontinued standard short-course therapy can lead to drug resistance, whether improved standard short-course chemotherapy can reduce the incidence of MDR TB and the epidemiological and economic impacts of poorly implemented DOTS programs both need to be evaluated (Dyer, 2002).

Tuberculosis is the leading cause of death for people with HIV/AIDS. In the past, interventions for TB and HIV/AIDS have been viewed and evaluated separately. Program evaluators need to establish norms and guidelines for evaluating the increasing number of "joint" programs for HIV/AIDS and endemic diseases and for addressing the measurement and evaluation challenges they pose (WHO, 2003a).

HIV/AIDS

The Joint United Nations Programme on HIV/AIDS (UNAIDS) estimates that in 2004 nearly 40 million persons were living with HIV and 3.1 million died from AIDS, about 95 percent of whom live or lived in developing countries. Perception of HIV/AIDs not as an isolated medical condition but one within a larger social context has important implications for the complexity of evaluation of HIV/AIDs programs.

At one level, the complex array of sociological factors that contribute to modes and rates of HIV/AIDs transmission generate substantial challenges in attribution, i.e., establishing the link between the intervention and individual HIV rates. Programs that indirectly affect viral transmission, such as HIV education programs, require robust evaluations that capture multiple elements along a lengthy, complex causal chain between intervention and disease burden. However, as researchers begin to appreciate the extent to which HIV's toll on society far surpasses disease rates through its leading toward greater economic and social upheaval, the impacts of evaluation shift from medical outcomes toward the larger societal goals of preserving the workforce, the family unit, and community function. This appreciation of the larger social and economic benefits of HIV prevention also provides additional incentives for investment in prevention programs.

When public health programs are operating in developing countries, the indirect effects generated by those programs may be less predictable than the effects in more-familiar Western settings. For example, a hypothetical vast mobilization of antiretroviral treatments (ARTs) for HIV patients could have substantial economic, political, psychological, and behavioral impacts far beyond those from a medical perspective. In terms of social impacts, the commitment and ability to treat HIV patients could have substantial impacts on (1) the stigma and fear associated with HIV, (2) native perceptions and distrust of Western activities in developing countries; (3) increased recognition of AIDS as a real disease (many birth certificates still record only the ultimate cause of death, such as tuberculosis).

In terms of economic impacts, the urgent needs of ART programs to train new staff to dispense medicines could generate a new class of rapidly trained clinicians. Keeping people sufficiently healthy to hold jobs, support their families, and keep their children in school could have vast economic implications. In terms of biological impacts, reducing HIV patients' viral load (the amount of HIV virus in an individual's blood stream) reduces the probability of additional infections and the chance of further viral transmission to children as well as to sexual partners.

The political effects could also be substantial, as national governments cooperate with international aid organizations on programs they both endorse, rather than on controversial condom-distribution and sexual-education activities. These effects are posed as hypothetical conjecture to illustrate the vast social context of HIV/AIDs and, as a result, the importance of taking these social and economic impacts into account when evaluating HIV/AIDs interventions.

Challenges Facing Program Evaluation

Interventions targeting diseases that can be prevented with vaccines and tuberculosis, malaria, and HIV/AIDS have unique characteristics that pose a number of specific challenges to program-impact evaluations. Interventions for vaccine-preventable diseases involve changing prevention behaviors, i.e., access to and acceptance of immunizations. Malaria does not have a clear prevention mechanism, it involves another vector (the mosquito), and it has multiple illness response mechanisms. Evaluating the impact of malaria-prevention interventions on both humans and the virus-host mosquito populations is relatively difficult. TB is difficult to diagnose, and there are few prevention mechanisms besides isolation and better economic and social conditions. An established treatment regimen (DOTS) has been implemented in many areas as a wide-scale social intervention that precludes using randomized controlled trials to identify cost-effective TB-treatment strategies. Unlike TB, HIV/AIDS is a chronic disease requiring lifelong care and with tremendous impact on families, communities, and developing countries. The interventions involve prevention, diagnosis, and treatment. While there have been systemic global immunization efforts for smallpox and other diseases that can be prevented with vaccines, the lack of a single effective prevention intervention (i.e., a vaccine) has led to endemic intervention responses for malaria, TB, and HIV/AIDS that, while globally informed, have been implemented on a local level.

Part of the rationale for program evaluation comes from the important role that monitoring and evaluation played during earlier immunization campaigns, such as the campaign for the global eradication of smallpox. The immunization campaigns lent themselves particularly well to a particular form of rapid evaluation of relatively easily measurable biological outcomes, which could be used to identify problem areas and quickly target resources. Determining program effects rapidly enabled researchers to prove small successes early on in the immunization campaigns, reversing the initial doubts of the donor community and government leaders and garnering needed support from important stakeholders.

While earlier immunization campaigns fed off a rapid feedback loop of information and assessment, current programs frequently outpace the level of knowledge needed to logically direct program efforts and to determine which programs really work. More-recent public health interventions have struggled to break out of the evaluation model set by the immunization campaigns to develop evaluation methods better suited to the more multidimensional epidemiology of diseases such as HIV and malaria, which require more-complex strategies for prevention, diagnosis, and treatment, and, therefore, require more-complex tools to assess the interventions for these diseases.

Evaluation of public-health interventions in developing countries is slowly evolving from process-focused monitoring of inputs, outputs, and expended funds toward more-scientific evaluation of long-term effectiveness and impact of the interventions. Scientific and ethical imperatives have placed pressure on public-health programs to demonstrate evidence of their effectiveness in developing countries, rather than simply relying on implicit policy assumptions about their effectiveness. There is increased recognition of the vast gaps in the knowledge that is needed to guide public health efforts, and at the same time, political controversy surrounds contentious issues such as provision of antiretroviral medications, use of DDT insecticide to combat malaria, and the appropriateness of sexual education and condom distribution programs for HIV prevention. When decision-makers are presented with a variety of evaluation options with varying costs and benefits, their selection of the most appropriate evaluation must be based on an understanding of the epidemiological issues surrounding the targeted disease and a strategic calculation of the scope of evaluation required to obtain useful information about the program's impact.

The primary purpose of an impact evaluation is to determine the net effect of an intervention. Interventions in all four public health areas—vaccination campaigns, HIV/AIDS, malaria, and tuberculosis—warrant a complete evaluation that captures both direct and indirect effects of a program within a given community. The relative magnitude of indirect versus direct effects inevitably will vary by intervention and by disease. As degrees of separation between intervention and medical outcomes increase, and as causal chains become weakened by confounding factors, the scope of an evaluation increases. Evaluators need to acquire a greater appreciation of the magnitude of indirect effects and develop better skills to measure those effects so that they can measure the real impact of interventions and inform policy debates and allocation of public health resources.

Study Approach and Methods

We undertook three basic activities in this study. First, we read peer-reviewed literature pertaining to program evaluation issues, both in general and with respect to health interventions in developing countries. We used this material as background information for preparing this report. Second, we reviewed evaluations of interventions for HIV/AIDS and TB in resource-poor countries to gain a better understanding of the rigor of impact evaluations in those countries. Our emphasis was on more recent evaluations so as to reflect the current state of practice. Finally, we convened a multidisciplinary team of RAND experts to discuss the methodological issues related to measuring the effects of complex health interventions.

The team also brainstormed over whether methodological approaches used in other disciplines might be used be used to address some of the methodological issues related to attributing measured effects to a health intervention (discussed in Chapter Three of this report). We found that the statistical techniques used to address the issue of attribution are well established. Although those techniques should be known to most health-services researchers, they have been used in evaluations of only a few notable health interventions in developing countries. Nevertheless, the number of evaluations employing those techniques is growing. However, the real issue is one of evaluative capacity—in terms of both expertise in recognizing the methodological issues and properly applying state-of-the-art measurement techniques and in having the resources to use those techniques.

Organization of This Report

Chapter Two establishes a conceptual framework for impact evaluations of health projects in developing countries. Chapter Three provides an overview of methodological and data issues related to evaluations of the indirect as well as direct effects of health interventions. Chapter Four reviews the current status of program evaluation of health interventions, using case studies for HIV/AIDS and TB in developing countries, and describes the Mexican government's PROGRESA national nutritional program as a "gold standard" for impact evaluation. Chapter Five identifies research and actions by funding organizations that would promote more-rigorous impact evaluations.

CHAPTER TWO

A Conceptual Framework for Evaluating Health Projects in Developing Countries

Traditional Framework for Program Evaluation

Program evaluation across all fields and disciplines is intended to (1) judge the effectiveness and worth of programs in order to maintain an ethical standard of accountability and (2) direct future program design so that resources are efficiently targeted to the most effective interventions and the groups that would benefit the most from those interventions. To accomplish these objectives, evaluation should take place throughout the various stages of an intervention, starting in the project-design phase with a baseline assessment and consideration of historical trends, and ending with an assessment of ultimate outcomes. At any given stage of the intervention, the focus, scope, and technical issues will vary depending on the intended purpose of the evaluation at that stage. Generally, a well-designed evaluative strategy involves various types of evaluations over the course of an intervention, including the following:

- **Formative evaluation.** A *formative evaluation* occurs when a project is first initiated. The purpose of the evaluation is to clarify objectives and to refine the project design, including the evaluation strategy and data requirements. Health interventions developed in one setting cannot simply be transferred across countries and cultures without making suitable adaptations (Hohmann and Shear, 2002). The basic principles of care may remain the same across cultures, but the actual strategies and programs for implementing important intervention principles must be tailored to the social and cultural needs of individuals and to the organizational and societal structures of their community. In considering these important issues, formative evaluations influence the choice of interventions and appropriate adaptations of those interventions.

An important aspect of formative evaluation is the collection of baseline data and historic data on pre-existing trends. Without appropriate and timely baseline surveys and trend estimations, it is difficult to argue for the effectiveness of any program. Whether comparing measures across locations or across time at a single location, the results may be biased if the underlying trends are not taken into account. The formative evaluation should also be used to design the post-implementation evaluation strategy of the intervention, including the methodologies, measures, and data requirements.

- **Process evaluation.** A *process evaluation* provides timely feedback on whether program administrators were able to carry out their activities according to plan. It provides information on how well the original plan was devised and what might be done to improve it operationally to achieve desired outcomes. Process evaluations support both monitoring activities and evaluation. *Monitoring activities* concentrate on structural inputs and processes, with some attention paid to project outputs. *Evaluation* focuses on outcomes and addresses the issue of program impact. The process evaluation findings can lead to improvements in program design and, just as important, support the impact evaluation by providing real-time data on how the intervention was carried out and whether it was implemented as intended. Process evaluations can also assess how the implementation mechanisms influence or distort the ability to achieve the final desired impacts (Maiorana et al., 2004).

- **Impact evaluation.** An *impact evaluation* assesses the overall impact of an intervention—whether it addressed its objectives and how it affected participating individuals and organizations, countries, and funders. Such evaluations examine both short-term program outcomes and longer-term system impacts. The question being asked—what impact did the project have?—requires an understanding of what the outcomes would have been without the intervention, holding all other factors constant. The impact evaluation informs funding organizations and policy decisionmakers on the decision whether to reinvest in or scale up a particular program.

If supported by a strong process evaluation, an impact evaluation provides information that can be used to design interventions in new sites that take advantage of the knowledge, experience, and lessons learned in similar cultural environments. By identifying particular components of the intervention that were critical to the project's success or failure, future program design can capitalize on lessons learned from an earlier project and avoid implementing the same intervention again when it is not possible or appropriate.

In a well-designed evaluative strategy, evaluation at each stage of a project informs the other stages. Traditionally, the bulk of evaluation occurs after a project has been implemented through process evaluation of inputs and outputs and some monitoring of outcomes. These process evaluations should create a feedback loop for continuous quality improvement in project design and implementation and also provide the information needed for the impact evaluation. Formative evaluations during the program-design stage and impact evaluations tend to receive less attention than process evaluations, yet both are extremely important in the context of health interventions in developing counties. Designing a successful intervention requires knowing what works well in a particular cultural environment and what issues are most likely to arise. What works well in one context may be ineffective or counter-productive in another context; therefore, culturally sensitive impact evaluations are needed. To inform future program-design decisions, the feedback loop in the evaluation model should include wide dissemination of findings from rigorous impact evaluations of health interventions in developing countries.

Scaling Evaluation Intensity to Potential Impact

Within the general model for program evaluation, various methodologies must be utilized selectively to develop and convey the information that is most pertinent to the goals and objectives of the particular project being evaluated. The challenge here is to develop an evaluative strategy that is most suitable to (1) the intervention's scope, design, and purpose; (2) its potential for being scaled up or replicated elsewhere; and (3) the potential value of the information that will be generated from the evaluation. The challenge is greatest when assessing health outcomes and system impacts of health interventions in developing countries, where the assumed benefits of many interventions remain unproven, and where methodological issues, evaluative capacity, data, and resource constraints make impact evaluations difficult.

Monitoring of inputs, outputs, and immediate outcomes is an evaluative strategy expected of nearly all projects and is needed for program accountability, continuing investment decisions, and program improvement. More-complex evaluative strategies address issues that cut across individual sites and/or examine long-term system impacts. These more resource-intensive evaluations are appropriate for a relatively small number of projects.

- The *common-outcomes evaluation* compares outcomes of similar projects, either for the same initiative in different sites or for interventions with similar objectives that are designed differently. This evaluation is helpful in identifying "robust practices," i.e., effective ways to achieve a particular objective that are likely to have applicability in other settings. The evaluation requires that there be common process or outcome indicators across the intervention sites, and it may necessitate additional data collection using common measures that allow cross-site comparisons.
- A *system impact assessment* focuses on the long-term effects of interventions. It typically follows or is done in conjunction with a common-outcomes evaluation. The evaluation questions should be defined by the strategic objectives for the health project and,

as discussed below, may extend beyond changes in health status and the health-care system infrastructure to more general political, social, and economic advancements. A scientifically rigorous, external evaluation is typically required to support findings about the efficacy or cost-effectiveness of a program.

Typically, the size and complexity of the evaluation matches the size of the project and is proportional to the amount of resources invested in the project. However, evaluation should not necessarily be proportioned according to project size, but perhaps more important, to the pre-existing level of evidence that is predictive of the project's effect, the significance of the disease burden, and the relevance of the intervention to policy.

Beneficial treatments must reach large numbers of individuals if global health goals are to be realized. Thus, the most valuable evaluations determine not only whether a program works but also whether a beneficial program may be successfully scaled up to a regional or national level. When previous evaluations have already conclusively established a link between a certain program and desired outcomes, subsequent evaluations may rely on practical assumptions, and it may be sufficient to limit evaluation to implementation rather than invest in re-confirming known links to outcomes. For example, vaccination campaigns often take advantage of well-established links between vaccination and disease prevention and include vaccination rates as surrogate indicators for health improvement, rather than direct measures of changes in disease burden.

Assessment of an intervention's long-term impact on a community's social and economic systems is most important when the links between activities, intermediate outcomes, and longer-term outcomes and system impacts are not well established by empirical evidence. Public-health success stories of the past, such as the smallpox eradication campaign, benefited from the short, direct link between vaccination and prevention of disease and relied heavily on real-time impact monitoring to provide immediate feedback to inform targeted efforts and provide evidence to justify scale-up. Diseases such as HIV and malaria, which continue to resist development of an effective vaccine, require preventive interventions that target upstream, often-causal pathways, such as sexual activity or exposure to mosquitoes. The more complex epidemiology of these multifaceted diseases requires more-sophisticated program evaluation techniques to capture their indirect causal pathways.

Policy decisions are inherently political, and efficacy or cost-effectiveness studies, even those that are highly precise, may or may not play a major role in the ultimate decisionmaking regarding intervention strategies. Nevertheless, even if the intervention design is pre-determined, or if the policy decision regarding whether to scale up must be made before the results from a pilot project are available, evaluation remains important. A formative evaluation is still needed to adapt the intervention design to the peculiarities of the culture or organization within which it will be implemented and to establish a baseline assessment and historic trends. A rigorous impact assessment would contribute to the evidence base for global health interventions and may lay the groundwork for policy changes based on evidence and for future interventions at another time or place. Further, large-scale implementation may have system impacts that are not evident at the pilot project level, and an impact assessment would contribute to the evidence base for global interventions and inform future policy decisions.

Using a Logical Framework to Stage an Evaluation

Public health evaluations in developing countries increasingly build on the *logical framework* (or "log frame") approach to monitoring and evaluation, which divides an intervention into stages, or "logical frames." The framework is used during the formative evaluation to clarify intervention objectives and to develop prospectively the causal chain linking inputs, outputs, intermediate outcomes, and the final outcomes. Indicators are developed for each stage of the intervention so that the key links in the causal chain are tracked and any exogenous factors are identified. Evaluation proceeds from one stage to the next only if the prior stage of indicators meets the required standards.

Using the log frame approach, time- and resource-heavy impact assessments are completed only upon prior demonstration of sufficient inputs and outputs to plausibly generate the desired outcomes. Most projects do not warrant an evaluation of the effectiveness of the final impact of their activities because the causal chain is broken at some point.

Three stages of post-implementation evaluation can be conceived using a prospective evaluation design:

Stage One

The first stage involves process evaluation, which assesses the content, scope, or coverage of the intervention, together with the quality and integrity of implementation. If the process evaluation finds that the project is not being implemented as planned (the right material and process inputs are missing and/or the desired outputs were insufficiently in evidence), there is little reason to go ahead with the evaluation of short-term outcomes, but improvements should be made in the intervention design (Andrews, 2004).

Stage Two

If progress is made at the process-evaluation stage, then the next phase—short-term outcome evaluation—can be attempted. For example, in the UNAIDS framework for indicator selection for HIV/AIDS prevention programs, HIV-related behaviors (along with knowledge, attitudes, and beliefs about HIV) have been considered to be outcomes. To be considered an outcome evaluation of the intervention's effectiveness, the link to causality would need to be well-defined and the nonintervention factors accounted for. If no positive changes occur in the short-term outcome measures, such as risky sexual or drug-taking behaviors, there is little point in going to the third phase of evaluation and looking at longer-term impact measures, such as HIV or sexually transmitted infection (STI) prevalence in the target population. (There would, however, be advantages to further evaluation to determine why the intervention did not work). If short-term outcome indicators plausibly are changing due to the intervention, an impact evaluation may be warranted, which could attribute long-term changes in HIV infection to a specific intervention. Poor anti-retroviral therapy adherence in a treatment program is a failure in the causal chain after the short-term outcomes have been achieved (such as the percentage of those presenting with HIV being given the first round of drugs) and can still reduce the ultimate impact of the treatment program or cause unforeseen negative effects, such as drug resistance in the local virus clade (virus strains with same common ancestor) (Hosseinipour et al., 2002). Thus, the impact assessment should determine not only whether the intervention was effective but also why it was or was not effective.

Stage Three

In a well-designed intervention with pre-existing trend data and a baseline survey, the monitoring of program data and surveillance of disease incidence or associated health indicators during the life of the intervention should provide enough information to fulfill the needs of the program-logic model. Changes in the trend data for disease prevalence and mortality when process and outcome indicators have been positive may be sufficient to suggest whether the intervention makes a difference.

The final phase of the evaluation then becomes the effectiveness study when the criteria for an impact evaluation are met. The advantage of such "prospective" impact evaluations—which are part of the design of the project itself from the beginning—is that the evaluation is a dynamic process that does not have to take the program implementation as given. If a process evaluation identifies problems with how the project is being implemented, changes can be made to the design and implementation to modify its processes, inputs, and outputs that would affect the ultimate outcomes. Another advantage of the prospective evaluation is that it can begin to trace program effects, regardless of where in the evolution of the health care intervention the evaluation begins.

There are, however, several potential disadvantages to "prospective" impact evaluations. First, there is a trade-off between making changes to improve the intervention and understanding why the intervention worked or did not work. Mid-course modifications in program design make it difficult to define what the intervention actually was and could hinder replication and scaling-up activities. Second, an evaluator's participation in each stage of the intervention could lead to the evaluator becoming "vested" in the project results. Third, the evaluator's participation may change the behavior of the project team in ways that otherwise would not have occurred (the "Hawthorne effect" [see Rossi, Freeman, and Lipsey, 1999]).

System Impact Assessments

The increased participation of general development organizations, such as the World Bank, in global health initiatives reflects an appreciation of the role of health as a critical component in overall economic development and nation building. These international organizations increasingly view improvement of global health not only as an end in itself, but as a stepping-stone for general economic revitalization of developing countries. Three of the eight Millennium Development Goals agreed upon at the 2001 United Nations (UN) Summit pertain directly to health: (1) reduce child mortality; (2) reduce maternal mortality; and (3) combat HIV, malaria, and other diseases. The motivation to alleviate the HIV epidemic in developing countries arises not only from the moral imperative to help sick people but also from an economic perspective that national progress requires a healthy population.

In order to prove that a given intervention generates final outcomes related to desired objectives, evaluations must establish the integrity of a logical chain of events linking observable changes directly caused by the intervention to downstream health changes observed in the population. When the objectives of global health initiatives are to stimulate overall development and economic growth, the endpoints for program evaluation are expanded beyond health outcomes to more general political, social, and economic advancements, or system impacts. Alleviation of disease as an intermediary objective toward improving larger national development requires expanding the scope of evaluation to measure impacts beyond changes in disease burden and diversifying the criteria by which public health programs are judged. Not only does evaluation utilize surrogates to measure health, but health itself becomes a surrogate for measuring general development, provided the link between improved health and economic development has been established in prior research. As the surrogate chain is stretched further from program activities to expansive development goals, the burden falls increasingly on evaluation to maintain the integrity of the chain (see Figure 2.1).

Funding organizations need to be realistic about the goals of and objectives for an intervention; however, if an organization's objectives include broad development goals, these goals should be explicitly examined as part of an evaluation. A pitfall in current evaluation is a persisting "disconnect" between the stated objectives of the sponsoring institution and what is measured in evaluation. Evaluation often considers incongruously narrow measures related to successful project implementation and does not take into account the outcomes and impacts relating to the intervention's broader goals and objectives. Evaluations of significant interventions should be framed to assess not only individual program success but also to provide information that pertains directly to the program's broader objectives.

Many program administrators assume that all improvements in health correspond to overall development goals, making the shift toward the endpoint of the evaluation continuum more a matter of semantics than an indication of any meaningful change in evaluation techniques. However, the presumed link between health outcomes and economic development goals often requires further investigation

Figure 2.1
Lineal Cause-and-Effect Model for System-Impact Assessments

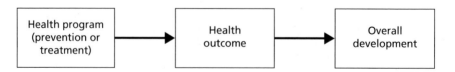

and methodologies that go beyond traditional program evaluation. Some health outcomes may serve as better indicators of general development than others. For example, prevalence rates for TB are affected by poverty and poor living conditions. Similarly, some desired outcomes in development may arise more from the capacity-building activities that are performed to achieve an intended health impact than from the health impact itself. Thus, health promotion activities may lead to overall advancements, whether or not the desired health outcomes are achieved.

Figure 2.2 depicts how health program activities may contribute to development goals, irrespective of the extent to which they produce intended intermediate health outcomes. For example, a program to treat HIV patients with ART may generate many outcomes regardless of whether patients are able to sufficiently adhere to stringent drug protocols to receive any medical benefit. In terms of health infrastructure, providing ART will require building numerous new clinics and recruiting and training many additional staff. Monitoring viral resistance will require additional lab capacities. The impact on the health infrastructure will depend on whether the additional capacity strengthens the overall health-delivery system or is achieved at the expense of other components of the delivery system. Politically, a country introducing ART may have to formulate new pharmaceutical importation and clinician licensing policies. In terms of social issues, the process of providing HIV patients with treatment may significantly reduce the social stigma associated with the disease, which in turn may encourage people to get tested or disclose their HIV-positive status. Even if reduction of viral load through ART does little to reduce population-wide transmission of HIV, the reduction may make HIV patients healthy enough to remain in the workforce or to care for their families, producing significant economic benefits.

Thus, if evaluators use only health outcomes as surrogate measures for overall development, they may miss a significant proportion of the potential impacts—positive and negative—of an intervention. As program operators face increasing pressure to prove favorable cost-benefit returns, comprehensive evaluation of the multiplicity of

Figure 2.2
Conceptual Framework for Evaluating an HIV/AIDS Intervention

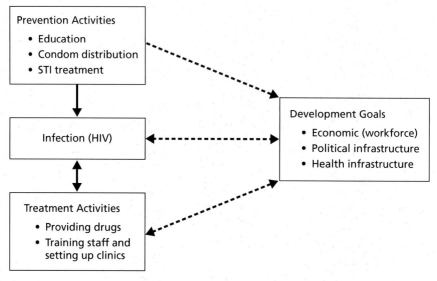

impacts conferred through program implementation becomes even more critical. However, comprehensive coverage of a highly complex web of social, medical, and economic inputs and outputs substantially increases the evaluation task.

CHAPTER THREE

Methodological Challenges in Evaluating the Impact of Health Projects in Developing Countries

This chapter primarily addresses the design of impact evaluations—the conscious and planned incorporation of evaluation needs into program design and implementation—so that both measurement and attribution of effects are more precise. The degree to which impact evaluations are useful and informative to decisionmakers depends on three factors: (1) the quality of the evaluation data and the precision with which the data are collected, (2) the magnitude of the effects, and (3) how much precision in measuring the effects is actually required for decisionmaking (the direction and magnitude of the effect may be more important than the preciseness of the estimate of the effect).

In the following sections, we provide a general overview of the methodological challenges in attribution and measurement. This overview is intended to highlight some of the major issues in gauging the effectiveness of health interventions and to serve as an underpinning for the later discussion of strategies that funding organizations might employ to increase evaluative capacity and the rigor of evaluations of health projects in developing countries. More detailed information on the evaluation issues and the techniques for addressing those issues can be found in the literature cited in this chapter.

At the outset of this study, we assumed that certain attribution and measurement challenges could be informed by methodologies used in other disciplines to address similar challenges. Through a brainstorming session with a multidisciplinary group of RAND researchers, we found, however, that while the challenges are significant, the techniques—both quantitative and qualitative—to address them are well established in the literature and ought to be known to health services researchers. There is, however, a significant gap between state-of-the-art best practice and actual practice in conducting impact evaluations.

Attribution Issues

The main goal of an impact evaluation is to produce a valid estimate of the impact of the policy intervention. Obtaining this estimate requires asking the following question: How do the observed changes in the observational unit (e.g., individual, family, community, or region) compare with the changes that would have been observed without the intervention, holding all other factors constant? Because one cannot directly measure what would have occurred without an intervention, a comparison must be made to a control group, or the evaluation model must otherwise incorporate statistical controls. Common statistical techniques to make such comparisons include the following:

- Randomized control trials that compare those individuals at an intervention site who were part of the intervention with those at the site who were not part of the intervention.
- Randomized cluster trials that compare populations at the intervention site with populations at a control site.
- Quasi-experimental designs that use non-random means to construct experimental and control groups.
- Pre- and post-regression analyses.

As discussed in the subsections that follow, the challenge in making these comparisons is to control for all other factors that might influence the estimate of the intervention's effectiveness. Choosing among evaluation design options requires making trade-offs. One approach to design selection is a "good enough" rule that selects the best methodological approach, taking into account the potential value of the evaluation results, feasibility of the design, and the probability of producing credible results (Rossi, Freeman, and Lipsey, 1999).

Internal and External Validity

To be useful, an impact evaluation should have both internal validity and external validity. *Internal validity*—the extent to which the evaluation results are reproducible using the same research design and setting—is determined by the power of the research design and is generally greater for randomized controlled trials than for other techniques. *External validity*—the extent to which the results are generalizable for similar interventions in the broader community or in other settings—is greatest if the intervention is implemented as it would be in the community.

It is not possible to conduct an experiment to test general conclusions for each local setting where an intervention might be implemented, which presents a unique problem for intervention design as it relates to effectiveness. Small, highly intensive programs designed to produce maximum outcomes in a particular location may replicate poorly at a larger scale in variable settings with looser control over implementation. A trade-off is often required between internal and external validity, and there is some debate among evaluators over whether internal or external validity is more important. One suggested approach is for researchers to emphasize internal validity when an intervention is first introduced in order to identify those interventions that are effective in at least some circumstances, and to stress external validity later to determine whether it will work under other conditions. When results from a large number of well-designed evaluations of similar interventions are available, meta-analysis can be used to examine systematically both internal and external validity (Rossi, Freeman, and Lipsey, 1999).

Unobserved Heterogeneity

A major challenge in assessing the impact of a social program is being able to "hold all other factors constant." The goal is to establish identical control and experimental groups, i.e., groups that are comparable in composition, predisposition, and experiences (Rossi, Freeman, and Lipsey, 1999). With identical control groups, any differences in effect can be attributed to the intervention. In social interventions, however, the pervasiveness of diversity among individuals means that unobserved heterogeneity between treatment and control groups is likely to persist. There will likely be unobserved heterogeneity between two groups unless the assignment of individuals within the population to the two groups is completely random. Such pre-existing differences between intervention and control group are known collectively as "selection bias." Selection bias occurs even within experiments with randomized selection among those who agree to participate in an intervention and may bias the evaluation results. The difficulty of identifying and extracting selection bias from an evaluation increases attribution of outcomes to the program itself, rather than to the composition of the group targeted for the intervention.

One way to reduce selection bias is to use "propensity score matching" to match individuals with similar probabilities of being treated during the intervention based on available observable characteristics. Alternatively, differences in observable characteristics that affect selection bias can be statistically controlled for using multivariate statistical techniques. The most sophisticated of these methods involves two-stage regression analysis in which the first stage models the selection bias, and the second stage uses the results of the selection bias regression as a predictor variable in estimating the effect of the intervention (Rossi, Freeman, and Lipsey, 1999). These methods of reducing selection bias rely on the correct identification of all potentially relevant variables. In the unfamiliar settings of developing countries, researchers may find themselves ill-equipped to identify critical differences among groups of people, further diminishing their ability to account for selection biases and possibly resulting in misleading inferences.

Randomized Control Trials

Researchers typically associate *randomized control trials* (RCTs) with the highly controlled efficacy studies performed on drugs and medical devices. However, the use of randomized designs in public-health trials does not attempt to extract confounding variables during the course of a study. Rather, the randomization attempts to make up for the fact that constellations of confounding variables cannot be fully accounted for through structural econometric approaches. Random assignment of the target population into an intervention or control group provides a powerful tool for ascribing different outcomes to the intervention itself and eliminating many potential selection biases. Although they have long been the gold standard of Western medical practice, until recently randomized trials generally have not been included in evaluations of public-health interventions in developing countries. As a practical matter, randomized trials are often more expensive to implement than quasi-experimental designs and require a long evaluation cycle involving substantial planning and implementation at the outset of a project (Rossi, Freeman, and Lipsey, 1999).

Well-designed and well-controlled randomized evaluations provide a means for averting statistical bias. Some potential biases are well-known and relatively feasible to measure. For example, evaluators may not have complete control over the random assignment of groups, individuals assigned to the treatment group may not ultimately participate in the program, or there might be contamination of the control group by random movement of people into and out of the treatment or control group. Unless assignment is completely random—i.e., individuals either elect to participate or are selected to participate in the pool from which the treatment and control groups are chosen—there should be controls for selection bias. Randomized designs also need to be sensitive to ethical considerations regarding the care provided to the control group and the selection of those that are assigned to the treatment group.

The Declaration of Helsinki (World Medical Association, various dates) addressed the issue of withholding care from a control group: "The benefits, risks, burdens, and effectiveness of a new method should be tested against the best current prophylactic, diagnostic, and therapeutic methods." The Council for International Organizations of Medical Sciences (CIOMS) subsequently stated that the standard of care need not be "the best current method" anywhere, but it should at least be an established effective intervention

(CIOMS, 2002). The Nuffield Council on Bioethics (2002) has broadened this issue further by suggesting the following:

Wherever appropriate, participants in the control group should be offered a universal standard of care for the disease being studied. Where it is not appropriate to offer a universal standard of care, the minimum standard of care that should be offered to the control group is the best intervention available for that disease as part of the national public health system.

Thus, the established ethical standards permit giving treatment to some people and not to others, as long as an equitable determination is made regarding who is eligible for the experimental treatment and who receives the standard care. However, in cases in which an intervention is known to have an effect, such as DOTS and ART, researchers may be reluctant to implement randomized designs if individuals are deprived of vital services in order to calculate the effectiveness of such services relative to standard care or to compare one intervention to another. In addition, randomizing individuals to treatment and control groups where there is a strong incentive for individuals assigned to a control group to seek out intervention treatment increases the likelihood that control individuals seeking treatment will cross-contaminate intervention and comparison groups. Nevertheless, there is a growing body of literature that indicates RCTs are feasible in developing countries (Duflo, 2003). For example, a recent study in Zimbabwe found that RCTS in school-based HIV prevention interventions that are designed to determine the effectiveness of adolescent reproductive health programs are feasible and acceptable, providing that the communities are properly involved and consulted (Cowan et al., 2002).

Cluster-Randomized Trials

Recent innovative adaptations of randomized designs for community-targeted interventions demonstrate a potential methodology to determine more credibly whether health interventions actually work. Pilot health interventions are beginning to adapt randomized designs to large-scale programs aimed at the community level, overcoming many perceived barriers to the interventions, including ethical issues regarding control groups, funding limitations for evaluation, and the inability to control numerous variables. Although many researchers and program administrators continue to struggle with the statistical adaptations required for randomization at a community level and the accompanying higher costs, a growing number of case studies demonstrate the potential for randomized designs to avoid many of the methodological pitfalls that confound evaluation of non-randomized programs and that weaken results.

In *cluster-randomized trials,* geographically associated and matched groups of individuals are randomly assigned to an intervention. Such trials compare entire groups of individuals, whether or not a given community received an intervention. Thus, these trials measure not only individual responses to treatment, but general community effects that arise from individuals receiving treatment. In theory, while individuals receiving treatment may demonstrate no statistically significant effect, significant impacts may be observed at larger community levels, especially for programs targeting infectious diseases, which are greatly affected by social conditions.

Cluster trials and RCTS face similar methodological challenges. Cluster trials must appropriately match baseline and trend characteristics of control and intervention communities, control for external confounding factors influencing one group but not others, control for unobserved heterogeneity, and select the most appropriate unit of analysis to optimize both internal and external validity. Cluster trials with overly restrictive exclusion criteria (such as omitting from a study those clinics with insufficient reporting capacity) sacrifice degrees of internal and external validity. While cluster-randomized trials provide an additional dimension of real-world sensibility to RCTs, poorly planned randomization using inappropriate units of analysis will generate equally weak and ineffective evidence or statistically biased estimates of effects.

Quasi-Experimental Designs

When a randomized trial is not feasible, comparisons may be drawn between an intervention group and a similarly matched group that did not receive the intervention. Such a comparison can provide information on the extent to which larger changes were particular to the intervention group and are likely to be associated with the program itself, or information on whether these changes reflected a broader societal trend affecting communities, regardless of whether they received the intervention. The problem with this type of analysis is that comparison groups often differ in terms of socioeconomic status, disease burden, motivation, and leadership, and the challenges of addressing selection bias are greater than those posed by RCTs (Duflo, 2003).

Pre-Post Regression Analyses

Pre-post regression analyses compare outcomes of individuals or groups after their exposure to a program against a prior set of data describing the same individuals or groups before the intervention. The underlying assumption is that no change would have occurred in the absence of the intervention. Or, if unrelated events did occur during the course of the program that may have significantly affected the results, final impact evaluation attempts to take into account such outside events through modeling. However, for many unanticipated behavioral and health-related changes, it is difficult to differentiate between program-related and independent events, and for this reason, a pre-post comparison is not recommended for partial coverage interventions (those that cover less than 80 percent of a population) where randomized or quasi-experimental techniques can be used to compare the treatment and control groups. However, for a full-coverage intervention for which an appropriate control group cannot be established, a well-constructed time-series analysis is an acceptable solution. A long time-series of data is needed to plausibly attribute outcomes to program impact, rather than to existing trends and natural fluctuations in the indicators. Such long-term data tend to be unavailable in developing countries, and retrospective surveys may be required to employ pre-post analyses. If there are differences in the intensity or timing of how a full-coverage intervention is implemented within the community, cross-sectional analyses with controls for other important differences may be preferable to the time-series analysis (Rossi, Freeman, and Lipsey, 1999).

Measurement Issues

Evaluations of health interventions in developing countries also face measurement challenges—i.e., defining what to measure, identifying valid indicators, testing and using the indicators in the field, and finally, validating and using the data for analysis. In the subsections that follow, we highlight some of the most important measurement issues that are encountered in outcome evaluations and impact assessments.

What to Measure

The issue of what to measure involves three key questions: (1) What scope of effects should be measured (downstream, horizontal, and upstream)? (2) What is the unit of observation (individual, household, or community)? and (3) What types of effects should be measured (biological and nonbiological)?

An underemphasized bias in measurement stems from the omission of potentially important impacts. An evaluation by the National Bureau of Economic Research (NBER) (Dow et al., 1995) of a tetanus vaccine intervention highlights the importance of identifying unexpected consequences—upstream, horizontal, and downstream—in measuring program effectiveness. NBER found that the reductions in infant mortality rates resulting from a neonatal tetanus intervention could not be accounted for by a decrease in neonatal tetanus alone. Upon further investigation, NBER found that the pregnant women who received tetanus vaccinations appeared to invest greater resources in their health and the health of their neonatal child than did women who did not receive the vaccinations, based on perceptions of an increased likelihood of survival through infancy. The researchers supported this interpretation with evidence that children whose mothers received the tetanus vaccine had significantly larger birth weights and a decreased probability of death at six months, which could be directly linked to the vaccination (Dow et al., 1995).

A systemic effect that is often omitted from impact evaluations relates to the disease-prevention benefits of treatment—generating increased demand for testing, decreasing the stigma associated with the disease, mobilizing communities, and importantly, reducing transmission (UN Millennium Project, 2004). These benefits are horizontal effects at the individual, family, and community level. There is a need to develop measures of the entire range of such disease-prevention outcomes and provide some tools for rapid assessment of these "prevention" payoffs from treatment.

Another systemic effect that is often neglected in impact evaluations relates to the cost at the epidemic level from poorly run interventions. For example, an HIV/AIDS treatment program that is poorly monitored (either due to cost constraints or the lack of affordable monitoring equipment and proper protocols) can lead to poor adherence to the drug regimen and the appearance of drug-resistant viral strains due to the wrong ART type being prescribed for the specific HIV clade (Kent et al., 2003; Sethi et al., 2004). Similarly, in areas where the malarial parasite *p. falsiparum* is still responsive to a particular anti-malarial agent, overuse as part of a malaria-treatment program would be inimical to disease-control targets. In MDR TB treatment, programs that are not careful in their initial mix of drugs may lead to bacteria developing wider resistance to an even greater mix of drugs. These negative program impacts should also be assessed and considered in the evaluation, either at the intervention project level or at the national or donor level.

When it comes to systemic effects, there is still some debate on the extent to which the focus of an evaluation should be on biological or nonbiological effects. For example, in the case of HIV/AIDs treatment, the question is whether it is more important to measure clinical outcomes—such as CD4 counts to determine the strength of an individual's immune system, viral loads indicating the amount of HIV in an individual's blood, and weight gain—or whether it is more important to measure how many treated individuals return to the workforce, show signs of improvement in their emotional well-being (and potential reduction in being stigmatized), or indicate heightened family cohesion, and other such outcomes. Although these nonbiological indicators may be difficult to quantify and rapidly assess, they constitute important returns on the investment in improving the quality of life of individuals with TB, AIDS, and other debilitating diseases with prolonged symptoms. The focus on quality-adjusted life years (or QALY, an indicator created to measure the quality and quantity of life) and disability-adjusted life year (or DALY, an indicator of the time lived without a disability and without time lost due to premature mortality) in cost-effectiveness analyses may not adequately capture the nonbiological effects. Conceptually, these important indicators are a mid-point measurement along a continuum that spans from individual biological outcomes to community-level nonbiological outcomes.

Program evaluators also need to think about establishing norms and guidelines to address the measurement and evaluation challenges that the increasing number of "joint" programs for HIV/AIDS and endemic diseases poses (World Health Organization, 2003a). Because of the co-morbidity of HIV/AIDS and TB, efforts have been made toward combined interventions and twin-disease-sensitive evaluations. TB programs involving DOTS reduce mortality among individuals with HIV/AIDs, as do prevention and prophylaxis of other endemic infections that are potentially fatal for immuno-compromised patients (Hosseinipour et al., 2002). Similarly, early initiation of ART can help prevent TB infections—averting up to 7.3 cases of TB per 100 patient-years overall (Badri, Wilson, and Wood, 2002). If these two types of TB programs have different sponsors, the question of "what to measure" is too often answered by which program's effectiveness is in question instead of by addressing the joint impact of both programs.

How to Measure

The most important "how to measure" issues are (1) the lack of baseline and trend data (see the discussion in the next subsection) and (2) the continuing tension between the need for standardized indicators and the need for measurement methods that are locally relevant and culturally sensitive.

Standardization of criteria and methods is critical to being able to make comparisons across interventions, but this critical need is often in conflict with the need to customize the measures to local settings. The early experience with efforts to standardize measures for

AIDS/HIV programs illustrates this point. The WHO/Global Program on AIDS in 1994 developed a standardized package that identified ten prevention indicators (PIs), known as *PI1–PI10*, using five different methods of data collection. Many countries have used the PIs for some time, adapting them to local circumstances. The PIs were meant to track trends, but they rarely have been measured repeatedly over time. The reason they have not been widely repeated is that they are often not relevant to local needs (UNAIDS, 2000).

On the other hand, the shortcomings of relying on locally developed indicators for evaluation were illustrated in a report on a "lessons learned" workshop on six ProTest pilot projects in Malawi, South Africa, and Zambia (World Health Organization, 2004). The WHO ProTest initiative was established in 1997 to develop a more coherent response to TB in settings with high HIV prevalence through collaboration between TB and HIV/AIDS prevention and treatment programs. Because of the nature of the intervention, indicators were developed locally in close collaboration with local stakeholders. Workshop participants noted two shortcomings in this approach. First, the various criteria and methodologies made cross-site comparisons overly complex. Second, energy was expended at the local level to create indicators for activities that could have been covered by standard indicators, e.g., HIV-prevention indicators developed by the UNAIDS-led international collaboration. The participants recommended that existing indicators should be used wherever possible and that a core set of indicators specific to TB/HIV activities be developed for future projects (World Health Organization, 2004).

The tension between standardized and local measures arises in part from the multiple functions of evaluation. As discussed in Chapter Two, the indicators used for monitoring and continuous quality improvement that measure resource use, activities, and immediate outcomes are generally project-specific. These indicators need to meet the needs of local program participants and may involve developing new indicators or modifying existing ones. For the higher-level evaluations—common outcomes evaluations and system impact assessments—a common set of indicators is needed. One way to resolve the tension between standardized and local measures at these levels is for funding organizations to require a core set of indicators while allowing the local sites to add additional indicators as appropriate to their needs for project-specific activities. This is the approach being taken in the Roll Back Malaria (RBM) initiative, in which the partners have selected five global indicators that should be used by all participants but allow all countries implementing RBM strategies to define additional indicators tailored to the local epidemiological situation and RBM priorities (UN Roll Back Malaria, 2005). As a contingency, the core set of indicators could also be considered for other projects, so that the data would be available should a cross-site comparison be desired after project implementation.

Disease-specific global indicators have been established for HIV/AIDS, malaria, and tuberculosis. However, for impact evaluations, greater standardization is needed for indicators and for simple, rapidly assayable survey methods to measure the nonbiological impacts of interventions, such as the ability to return to work, family cohesion, and other such impacts. Nonbiological impacts are sensitive to the contextual environment of intervention—social, geographical, and ethnographic. For example, reduced social stigma may not occur in a given setting for an individual with HIV/AIDS, even when the individual is able to function with ART, and the ability to work may be meaningless in a zone of widespread unemployment. But even clinical issues vary by geography, ethnicity, and type of HIV clade infection. The sensitivity of ARTs' effectiveness to non-adherence, the barriers to adherence that are intrinsic to ART and HIV treatment, and the barriers to adherence found particularly in resource-poor settings all mean that close attention should be paid to local effects when measuring the impact of treatment interventions. Community and individual factors that affect an HIV/AIDs patient's adherence to ART include substance abuse, gender, age, mental health, education, success of first stage of ART, system of care, and provider-patient relationships (Kent et al., 2003). Therefore, measuring ART adherence with recognition of the contextual situation and allowing for the bias in self-reported adherence in assessing the effectiveness of an ART intervention are important areas for future evaluation research.

Data Limitations

We concentrate on HIV/AIDS in this discussion of data limitations because of the multifaceted nature of the disease and its relatively recent emergence; TB, malaria, and vaccine-preventable diseases have been tracked for a longer period than has HIV/AIDS.

Currently, the main sources of international data on HIV/AIDS in developing countries can be found in the following datasets: Demographics and Health Survey (DHS+), Reproductive Health Survey (RHS), World Development Indicators, Multiple Indicator Cluster Survey (MICS), Behavioral Surveillance Survey (BSS), and UNAIDS General Population Survey (see Appendix A) (USAID et al., 2005). The surveys vary widely in terms of how long they have been in the field. DHS+ and RHS have been in the field the longest and are still in use; however, HIV/AIDS data were not included in the early collection efforts, so limited trend data are available from these surveys. For example, the DHS was first implemented in 1984 but did not add an HIV/AIDS module until the early 1990s (Boerma and Sommerfelt, 1993). The addition of an HIV/AIDS module to the DHS coincided with other efforts to collect HIV/AIDS data in developing countries, beginning roughly in the late 1980s. The most comprehensive data available about the disease are still based largely on estimates.

Of these surveys, BSS and the UNAIDS General Population Survey collect data specific only to HIV/AIDS. HIV/AIDS-related indicators present in most, or all, of the data sets focus on condom availability and quality, social stigma and discrimination, knowledge of HIV/AIDS, voluntary counseling, mother-to-child transmission, sexual negotiation and attitudes, sexual behavior, injection-drug testing, drug use, blood safety, STI care and prevention, HIV/AIDS care and support, health and social impact from the disease, HIV/AIDS incidence, HIV/AIDS prevalence, and spending on HIV/AIDS programs (USAID et al., 2005).

While these surveys do share many common variables, definitions for various measures may not be uniform across all surveys. The surveys may differ over time as additions and modifications are made. The surveys may also vary between countries, thus decreasing cross-country comparability. For example, in the DHS+, time references for sexual behavior differ from those of the other surveys, and three time trends emerge: the past year, past six months, or past four weeks. Also complicating trend-data analyses are changes to wording or sequencing of survey questions over time (USAID, 2002). The lack of standardized definitions poses a challenge to accurately understanding the state of the HIV/AIDS epidemic. Further limitations to interpreting similar data from multiple sources include differences in the frequency of collection efforts and the time lag from data collection to publication of results.

These data are intended for surveillance. While they have the potential to measure systemic change at the national level and in some cases the subpopulation level, they generally do not support project-level impact evaluations that require small-area data for baseline data, cross-site and population comparisons, and trend lines. Data collection is a major cost driver for impact evaluations. Consequently, when resources are limited, resource allocation choices may need to be made between funding to support surveillance and capacity-building for national monitoring and evaluation, and funding for data collection needed to conduct impact evaluations. To the extent appropriate, administrative data that are already being collected for monitoring and surveillance should be utilized so as not to burden the program more than necessary. Ultimately, investments in the data infrastructure and prospective data collections on the geographic reach of interventions, risk-population coverage, inputs, intensity, and the characteristics and activities of the interventions will support not only evaluation of specific programs but also enhance national monitoring and evaluation systems (MAP, 2002).

Use of Surrogate Markers

Surrogate markers serve as essential shortcuts to drawing logical connections within a complex web of interrelated factors. When direct measurement is infeasible or unpractical, evaluation inherently entails the rational utilization of surrogate measures based on statistically credible associations to draw indirect connections between program activities and objectives and goals farther downstream. Surrogates are commonly used as proxy measures for outcomes that may be infeasible to quantify or difficult to measure. For example, because many factors affect HIV rates, HIV condom-distribution programs may base evaluations on surveys of condom use rather than measure the ultimate desired outcome of reduction in HIV rates. The surrogate is not only easier to measure than the reduction in HIV rates, but it is also easier to attribute directly to an intervention. While the link between the intervention and the surrogate may be strong, the link between the surrogate and desired outcomes may vary. For example, the contribution of population-wide increases in condom use to the ultimate reduction in the HIV burden remains a controversial issue.

Just as scientists continually experiment with different biological markers to determine which is most strongly linked to a disease of interest, program evaluators must judiciously select surrogate markers with clearly established links to the desired outcome. The decision to use surrogate measures must be strongly guided by an informed understanding of the strength of assumed connections between surrogate measures and desired outcomes. Many surrogates have not been adequately tested across the diverse conditions of developing countries. In addition, general unfamiliarity with the culture and society of developing countries often renders the assumptions underlying surrogate markers more tenuous. Also, as health interventions increasingly attempt to target root causes of complex diseases arising from long causal chains of events, distances between surrogate measures and desired health outcomes become increasingly stretched.

The presumed links between surrogate measures and desired public-health outcomes in developing countries have undergone increased scrutiny in recent years. Controversial studies increasingly undermine conventional wisdom concerning the real benefit of current intervention strategies. For example, two studies (Todd et al., 2003; Orroth et al., 2003) conducted in similar settings along the Uganda-Tanzania border found conflicting results as to whether treatment of STIs reduced the transmission of HIV. Debate continues as to why these two studies had different findings. Regardless of which results better reflect the general contribution of STI treatment programs to HIV prevention, the growth of studies that challenge the presumed conventional wisdom regarding use of surrogate markers will clarify which markers hold up to scientific scrutiny and which assumptions require reevaluation. To determine the validity of presumed surrogates, such studies must recast the focus of program goals toward determining what really works, rather focusing purely on health outcomes.

Multidisciplinary Measures

Ideally, meaningful assessment of a project's impact in medical, economic, social, and psychological terms requires the joint collaboration of specialists from all of these fields. Moreover, the integration of public health with other academic fields stimulates a valuable exchange of evaluation methodologies and approaches. Yet, incorporating and synthesizing information from multiple academic disciplines into a coherently integrated analysis remains a significant challenge to multidisciplinary evaluation. Implicit understanding of rather esoteric terminology within disciplines makes it difficult for researchers in other disciplines to successfully utilize borrowed data and to accurately assess program impact across different dimensions. On a smaller, more practical scale, simple clarification of how social scientists arrive at their calculations, what those figures really mean, and how they might be used in health policy could greatly improve efforts of project evaluators to provide more comprehensive impact assessments.

If information produced through evaluation is to be useful, the terminology used to convey it must be clear and understandable outside of one's immediate field (Murray, 2003). Many researchers specializing in a specific field may be unfamiliar with the descriptions of evidence from other fields and with the degrees of uncertainty associated with external data. Blind use of figures calculated by experts in other fields could lead to misuse of the data and problematic disregard for degrees of uncertainty. For example, economists often use United Nations Population Division data on child mortality and life expectancy in their evaluations of which intervention strategies work. However, the UN often calculates these figures using models that relate income and education levels to child mortality and life expectancy, resulting in a perpetual cycle of reusing borrowed data and seriously biasing data. Likewise, evaluations by public-health analysts often rely on income per capita in international dollars to determine purchasing power, whereas economists often base purchasing power parities on regression models. Both of these examples demonstrate how information intended to guide strategic decisionmaking in one study can become misapplied in subsequent studies.

CHAPTER FOUR

Current Status of Program Evaluation in Developing Countries

Some notable high-quality evaluations demonstrate the value of rigorous impact assessments, such as the evaluation of Mexico's PROGRESA national nutritional program, described later in this chapter. However, our review of the literature and selected evaluations indicates that despite the acknowledged benefits of randomized studies, the great majority of evaluations continue to use standard regression methodologies.

For the most part, there is a considerable gap between best practices in program evaluation and actual practices in evaluative strategies. For example, the literature contains many analyses and reviews that address the methodological issues associated with cluster-randomized studies. Despite discussion in the literature of those issues and the availability of statistical tools and software to evaluate cluster-randomized studies, an evaluation of cluster-randomized controlled trials in sub-Saharan Africa (Isaakidis and Ioannidis, 2003) found the quality of the studies to be very poor. Only 20 percent of the studies took clustering into account for determining initial sample size or making power calculations during the planning stages of a program; only 37 percent took clustering into account in the final analysis; only 2 percent reported intracluster correlation coefficients; and only 6 percent described design effects. While Isaakidis and Ioannidis observed that the quality of analysis improved somewhat in studies after 1996, the dearth of reported data makes these studies difficult to interpret, analyze, and compare with other studies.

In the sections that follow, we first summarize our findings from a review of selected evaluations and several peer-reviewed surveys of evaluations—whether prospective or retrospective—which were not just baseline surveys or pilot programs. Our objective was to get a sense of the scope and quality of current evaluations in "resource-poor" settings, which we define as any country except countries belonging to the Organization for Economic and Cooperative Development (OECD) or countries with a real per-capita annual income of more than $10,000. For HIV/AIDS, evaluations of HIV/AIDS prevention, preventing mother-to-child transmission (PMTCT), and voluntary counseling and treatment (VCT) interventions were selected; for TB, evaluations for interventions other than drug efficacy trials were included. Our emphasis was on more recent evaluations, so as to reflect the current state of practice.

We conclude with an overview of the PROGRESA nutritional program and its evaluation, which is a model for the amount of influence a well-designed program can have on public policy.

Summary of Findings from the Review of HIV/AIDS Program Evaluations

A search of the National Library of Medicine PubMed database (at http://www.ncbi.nlm.nih.gov/entrez/query.fcgi?DB=pubmed), which tracks peer-reviewed life-science journals, using the keywords "HIV" and "evaluation," found a very small sample of evaluations or reviews of evaluation studies that fit the selection criteria discussed in the beginning of this chapter. Two reviews of previous evaluations provide a snapshot of the state of program evaluation: Scotland et al. (2003) for PMTCT (preventing mother-to-child transmission) programs in sub-Saharan Africa and Gallant and Maticka-Tyndale (2004) for school-based HIV/AIDS prevention programs. In addition, we found some individual evaluations from other sources. The relative lack of good, recent evaluation studies in the PubMed database, other than clinical trials for interventions in developing countries, is itself a cause for concern.[1]

Scotland et al. (2003) reviewed the methods and findings of studies that assessed the costs and consequences of PMTCT interventions in sub-Saharan Africa. The questions that the authors used as selection criteria for the economic studies demonstrate the key issues in review of evaluation studies:

- Study design: Is the research question stated?
- Effectiveness estimate: Are data source(s) for the estimate stated? Are primary outcome measures clearly stated? Are methods for the estimation of quantities and unit costs described?
- Analysis and interpretation of results: Is the choice of variables for sensitivity analysis justified?

Scotland et al. found nine studies that used modeling techniques to predict the cost-effectiveness of ART interventions. Their key findings on the design and quality of the evaluations were as follows:

- There was a lack of detail regarding the resources required for interventions and the methods for valuing health outcomes and unit costs.
- The generalizability of the findings was limited by the use of incremental costing and uncertainty regarding the level of infrastructure needed to implement the interventions. The models also suffered because the parameters were based on some assumptions made by the evaluators as well their subjective views.
- All but two interventions were evaluated only from the perspective of the ART provider. The exceptions also analyzed the patient's lost productivity as an indirect cost of HIV infection.
- Most studies depended on previously published results from the relevant randomized clinical trials (RCTs) to model the efficacy

---

[1] Additional searchable databases for a more exhaustive literature review include MEDLINE, EMBASE, AIDSLINE, OVID, abstracts of previous AIDS conferences, and hand searches of print journals (e.g., *AIDS, Journal of AIDS*).

of a particular drug in reducing transmission rates. Standardization may or may not be appropriate in all cases, considering the geographic and ethnographic variations in clinical results on drug efficacy and clinical practice across regions.

• Not all impacts were considered. For example, cost and survival trade-offs between reduced infant-HIV infections and greater numbers of AIDS orphans (who have lower survival rates in sub-Saharan Africa than in other parts of the world, according to the authors) were not considered. The costs and consequences to the mothers were also ignored, reflecting the reality of VCT in sub-Saharan Africa, where there are few resources available for infected mothers.

Several recommendations made by Scotland et al. are applicable to a wide range of HIV/AIDS evaluations:

• Prospective (economic) evaluations designed to run alongside pilot programs or RCTs are needed. The full costs and quantities of all the resources used by the intervention (including existing infrastructure) should be included, so that the results are more generalizable to other settings in sub-Saharan Africa.

• Models should be made more comprehensive by including more societal costs and consequences.

• Future research should be conducted in areas where there is uncertainty surrounding the parameter values used in economic models.

Gallant and Maticka-Tyndale (2004) reviewed 11 published evaluations of school-based HIV/AIDS risk-reduction programs for youth in Africa. Most evaluations were quasi-experimental designs with pre-test/post-test assessments. The program objectives varied. Some targeted only knowledge, while others targeted attitudes, and still others considered behavioral change. Gallant and Maticka-Tyndale provide details about the programs and identify characteristics of the most successful programs. Clearly, however, more research is needed to identify with certainty the factors that drive successful school-based HIV/AIDS risk-reduction programs in Africa.

In addition to Scotland et al. and Gallant and Maticka-Tyndale, we selected other recent evaluations for review, which are summarized in Table 4.1. The results were mostly disappointing except for an exceptional evaluation conducted in Kenya of a behavioral-change program using the WHO's clinical stages, which are widely used in modeling disease progression in treatment programs. The design for this cross-sectional evaluation is a benchmark for quasi-experimental evaluation of prevention programs.

Summary of Findings from the Review of TB Program Evaluations

A search on PubMed using the keyword set "tuberculosis" and "evaluation" and the keyword set "DOTS" and "evaluation" yielded some evaluations and one review of evaluations (studies of prevalence or drug resistance were excluded). Several problems remain in evaluations of DOTS interventions compared with the previous nonobserved (or poorly administered) treatment regimes. As Davies (2003) points out, the "gold standard" in evaluation of RCTs for TB interventions remains problematical, because as soon as the study begins, even patients in the control group (receiving non-directly observed treatment) receive better care than the care they received prior to the study. Poor handling of some issues of concern remains another issue for evaluations of DOTS in the developing world. For example, Pope and Chaisson (2003) surveyed three developing-country RCTs of the DOTS method and focused on treatment completion. They concluded that the RCTs were not comparable because of the different ways in which DOTS was operationalized (often failing to match the World Health Organization's definition for DOTS, as listed in under "Tuberculosis" in Chapter One).

Table 4.1
Summary of Selected Evaluations of HIV/AIDS Treatment Programs

Authors/ Year/ Location	Evaluated Area	Type of Design	Baseline or Pre-test	Sampling/ Quantitative Analysis	Quality of Attribution/ Conclusions
Kakande and Bunyole, 2004, Uganda	Prevention, care, orphan programs	Qualitative (focus groups) and survey	No	Purposive cluster sample (= 200),[b] HIV/AIDS knowledge polled	Results: Increase in program "awareness" and number served; attribution suspect; not rigorous
Harms et al., 2004, Kenya, Tanzania, Uganda	PMTCT programs. Donor: GTZ[a]	Cost evaluation per impact unit	No	Categorized costs, modeled results based on program results and assumed or standardized clinical results	Results: cost per infection prevented (Uganda); did not include broader costs; did not attempt broader impact analysis
Kassa et al., 1999, Addis Ababa, Ethiopia	WHO HIV staging system field test	Cross-sectional cohort study	Yes	Analysis of samples, correlation analysis, statistical matching	Results: WHO "clinical stages" work: match well with CD4-positive counts and viral loads; rigorous analysis
Jaratsist, 2004, Bangkok, Thailand	AIDS case reporting system	Qualitative analysis (interviews) and analysis of administrative records	No	Process analysis of case reports at various levels, matching of data, field interviews	Results: Basic process evaluation, reduced scope; intervention needs to be monitored over time for impact

Table 4.1—Continued

Authors/ Year/ Location	Evaluated Area	Type of Design	Baseline or Pre-test	Sampling/ Quantitative Analysis	Quality of Attribution/ Conclusions
Shantha et al., 2004, Chennai, India	Hospital VCT service	Hospital-record analysis, patient surveys	No	Data analysis of registers for number of repeat visits to the VCT supplemented with satisfaction surveys	Results: Repeat visits were taken as main proxy for success; no analysis of clinical outcome or impact; not rigorous
Erulkar et al., 2004, Kenya	Behavior change in a reproductive health program	Quasi-experimental design with comparable control	Yes	Cross-sectional surveys at baseline and endline, with some probability sampling; multivariate analysis of results (behavior indicators based on survey answers, personal details)	Results: Improved in all indicators; variables associated with adverse behaviors identified; study corresponds to best practices for data collection, design, and analysis; approaches attribution near RCT quality; rigorous

[a] Gesellschaft für Technische Zusammenarbeit, a German technical cooperative.
[b] A purposive sample is subjectively selected by a researcher. The researcher attempts to obtain a sample that appears to be representative of the population and will usually try to ensure that a range from one extreme to the other is included.

With these issues in mind, we also reviewed seven individual studies from 2001–2004 spanning a wide geographical range, which are summarized in Table 4.2. Recurring problems in the DOTS evaluations were the lack of a comparison with a pre-DOTS cure (i.e., a baseline measurement) and lack of data on sputum conversion and completion rates. Historical RCT studies show mixed results in finding DOTS the better treatment regime when compared with a placebo and with a limited sequence of other drug regimens,[2] and are also open to the sort of criticism that Davies (2003) levies. However, DOTS RCTs are still rare in developing countries. Within the DOTS sphere itself, the seven more-recent studies we reviewed showed that results can vary based on whether DOTS is administered by community volunteers, government health workers, or family members.[3] In fact, rates of adherence to therapy and completion of the prescribed course of treatment vary in particular.

Given that these variations in DOTS exist in practice and the evidence that these variations matter, evaluations should be specific in reporting the type of DOTS. The evaluations should also present completion rates prior to the start of an intervention, or other baseline results for comparison to what has been achieved in sputum conversion or completion rates at the end of the particular type of DOTS in question. Also, nonclinical outcomes and patient self-assessment of wellness can supplement the assessment of effectiveness of the treatment and the patient's tolerance of the regimen imposed by the particular DOTS type. A possible addition to cost-effectiveness studies of DOTS is an analysis of the benefits of averted treatment costs, but consideration of these benefits is not widespread. Many of these improvements in evaluation practice may require further standardization and development of field toolkits for rapid assessment of the effectiveness of DOTS interventions in developing countries (similar to the rapid assessments for HIV/AIDS treatment) (Floyd, 2002).

---

[2] See Zwarenstein et al. (1998) and Walley et al. (2001). Among non-RCT studies, see Norval et al. (1998) for a positive finding on DOTS.

[3] See Wright et al. (2004) and Lewin et al. (2005).

Table 4.2
Summary of Selected Evaluations of TB Treatment Programs

Authors/ Year/Location	Evaluated Area	Type of Design	Baseline or Pre-test	Sampling/ Quantitative Analysis	Quality of Attribution/ Conclusion
Miti et al. 2003, Zambia	DOTS short-course via home-based care for people living with HIV/AIDS (PLWHA)	Prospective quasi-experimental design with comparable control group	Yes	All new TB-positive cases in both groups; two-month sputum smear conversion and eight-month treatment outcomes studied	Results: Cure rate higher in home-based care group, lower treatment interruption Design: rigorous, attribution good
Ngamvithayapong et al., 2000, Chiang Mai, Thailand	Isoniazid Preventive Therapy (IPT) for latent TB in PLWHA	Retrospective cure-rate analysis, supplemented with interviews	No	71 hospitals reporting and 6 site visits; data inconsistency occurred (instrument not field tested)	Results: Poor outcome of IPT therapy, case load management poor, active TB should be referred to DOTS Design: not rigorous, poor data management
Adatu et al., 2003, Uganda	DOTS short-course option community supervision or Community-Based DOTS (CB-DOTS)	Retrospective quasi-experimental design, using same group as pre-post control group	Yes	Unequal pre-post groups; measured treatment success (cure), deaths, and treatment interruption rates; acceptability measured by survey of patients	Results: Treatment success increased, interruption declined; no significant change in death rate; acceptability was higher for CB-DOTS Design: Quite rigorous, included an evaluation of acceptance

Table 4.2—Continued

Authors/ Year/Location	Evaluated Area	Type of Design	Baseline or Pre-test	Sampling/ Quantitative Analysis	Quality of Attribution/ Conclusion
Singh et al., 2004, North India	Volunteer-based DOTS	Post-intervention comparison	No	Comparison of treatment success rate for volunteer-based DOTS versus DOTS with government health workers	Results: Found treatment success rates to be comparable Design: Poor rigor, no baseline; did not evaluate treatment interruption or mortality; no patient interviews to supplement findings
Nateniyom et al., 2004, Thailand	DOTS in prison population	Prospective analysis of program outcome, no control	No	1,412 consecutively occurring cases of TB in prison inmates, with TB-positive smear tracked for cure rate	Results: DOTS could not achieve national targets in cure rate Design: Isolated population excuses the lack of control; however, baseline needed

Table 4.2—Continued

Authors/ Year/Location	Evaluated Area	Type of Design	Baseline or Pre-test	Sampling/ Quantitative Analysis	Quality of Attribution/ Conclusion
Ruohonen et al., 2002, Leningrad, Russia	DOTS intervention supported by Finnish Lung Association	Retrospective case data analysis	No	859 TB cases (292 smear-positive) in Leningrad region tracked	Results: DOTS chemotherapy led to 71.3% treatment and 11.7% interruption rates Design: Without a baseline, it is difficult to say if this is an improvement or not
Kazeonny et al., 2001, Orel Oblast, Russia	DOTS short-course	Prospective case data analysis	No	570 patients enrolled from October 1999–March 2000 in two batches	Results: Treatment success of 81% and fatality of 12% among TB-smear–positive patients Design: Not rigorous; also, the effect of low rate of MDR-TB in the presented cases should be allowed for

Discussion of Findings from HIV/AIDs and TB Program-Evaluation Reviews

Our limited review indicates that designing an effective evaluation remains a problem for projects that are run in resource-poor settings. Even in well-designed evaluations with an external evaluator, the impact analysis is rarely broad enough to give a detailed view of societal impacts or secondary outcomes of an intervention. Given cost constraints, the lack of detail might be excused. However, the use of standardized parameters or previous study results for modeling effectiveness in the absence of persistent monitoring of the intervention in question suggests that insufficient attention is being paid by the program evaluators to the possible use of simple clinical markers, such as anemia, lymphocyte count, 1,500 cells per cubic millimeter of fluid, low body-mass index, and HIV/AIDS symptoms, which have been shown to be predictors of short-term survival. This is relevant for those situations in which other measurements for monitoring HIV/AIDS disease stage are not affordable. Similarly, for treatment effects, alternatives to CD4 counts exist, such as the defendable use of total lymphocyte counts (Van der Horst, 2002).

For the least rigorous evaluations, which typically lack sufficient funds and local evaluation expertise, there is a real opportunity to improve evaluation practice—for example, through the training of program evaluators and dissemination of easy-to-use tools for logic models, inexpensive long-term monitoring of clinical markers for resource-poor settings, and a baseline that ensures that effectiveness can be measured and attributed to the intervention to as high a standard as is reasonable (Ainsworth, 2004). For external, evaluator-led (and ostensibly rigorous evaluations), more attention needs to be given to indirect effects of the interventions (especially family and societal); the feasibility and applicability of RCTs should be considered (consistent with recommendations made by Cowan et al., 2002); some monitoring and surveillance capability should be ensured; and local evaluative support should be recruited to ensure sustainability of the post-program efforts so that impacts remain measurable in the longer term (Sallet et al., 2004).

The PROGRESA Program: A Case for Impact Evaluation

The Mexican government's PROGRESA national nutritional program provides a good example of how savvy administrators turned budgetary constraints imposed by the Mexican government into a robust evaluation scheme to rationalize further program scale-up. Unable to implement the public-health intervention nationwide from the start, the program managers introduced the program to randomly selected communities and compared outcomes in those communities with outcomes in matched, nonparticipating communities. The evaluation provided solid evidence of significant health gains in a range of various measures for communities enrolled in PROGRESA relative to the comparison communities; the evaluation also provided evidence of the overall cost-effectiveness of the program. The results provided grounds for expanding PROGRESA into additional communities.

In this regard, PROGRESA serves as a model for how public-health planners actually capitalized on the financial challenges posed by a developing country to devise a randomized evaluation design. Although the randomized evaluation design temporarily excluded certain communities from the benefits conferred by the program, the strength of the evidence generated by the evaluation design won the political support and financial backing needed to ultimately sustain and expand the program for the long-term benefit of all Mexicans. PROGRESA demonstrates how superior evaluations can serve as effective tools for identifying successful pilot programs worthy of scale-up. The element of randomization in particular justified the scale-up by proving that the program conferred benefits not only to specifically selected communities, but to any random community, suggesting greater generalizability of success to a variety of settings.

When the Mexican government began a national program linking school attendance to nutritional and preventive-health program benefits, budgetary constraints prevented the intervention from reaching all 50,000 potential beneficiary communities initially. Mindful that the continued government funding needed for scale-up, especially in the event of a likely regime change, would depend on evidence of initial program success, the government capitalized on this limitation by initiating a pilot phase of the program in which 506 randomly selected communities received the program. Baseline data on nutritional impact were collected from a random selection of communities during the intervention.

An independent group of academic researchers from the International Food Policy Research Institute (IFPRI) conducted the evaluation. Comparisons between beneficiaries and non-beneficiaries demonstrated that children receiving the intervention experienced 23 percent less illness, a 1–4 percent increase in height, and an 18 percent reduction in anemia. Enrollment of students in grades one through eight increased by 3.4 percent, and adults lost 19 percent fewer workdays due to illness (Rivera, 2004). Based on such evidence, the PROGRESA program did in fact survive turnover in the Mexican government. It reached 2.6 million families by 2000 (10 percent of all Mexican families), with a budget of $800 million (which represented 0.2 percent of the Mexico's gross domestic product in 2000), and was granted additional loans by the World Bank for scale-up. Having observed the power of evaluation to sustain political support, several Latin American countries have modeled similar programs after PROGRESA.

The PROGRESA example also demonstrates the role evaluation can play in scaling up from pilot programs. One of the great frustrations with generating large-scale national and regional health changes is that programs that are highly effective at the small pilot-program level with high-intensity implementation and that are tailored to local needs often prove to be less effective when scaled up to reach larger national and regional numbers. Randomized selection of intervention groups limits the extent to which programs will be fit to the specific needs of a single community. Randomizing pilot programs across a wide geographical area serves to better evaluate program impacts across a variety of contexts, increasing generalizability of findings.

PROGRESA also represents the increasingly multidisciplinary approach to public health as a field working in concert with other fields to address the issue of global poverty. Global organizations commit to not only alleviating specific disease burdens but also to promote the general well-being of impoverished populations. The PROGRESA program spans the economics, public health, and education fields by tying health-care packages and nutritional supplements to children's attendance at school and by providing conditional cash transfers for food and school supplies. The field of public health increasingly is seen as a fusion between medical biology and social science, which challenges program evaluations to assess a mix of economic, social, and medical variables using methods that fuse analytical techniques from all of these fields.

The PROGRESA program's scale-up protocol also demonstrates how ethical issues arising from depriving control communities of potentially beneficial services can be mitigated by following a phased-in introduction of a program, so that control groups eventually receive the same treatment as the original intervention group. In addition, by maintaining randomization throughout the incremental scale-up of the program, the effects of expanded operational levels on program outcomes could be tracked. Thus, researchers could continually evaluate the success of the scale-up as it proceeded and detect any effect of expansion on program impacts.

The PROGRESA program demonstrates that relatively simple designs thoughtfully and logically devised can greatly improve the quality and ultimate utility of evaluations to demonstrate real program success and can earn support for further expansion to benefit the broader population. PROGRESA reflects a growing optimism regarding the feasibility of rigorous evaluation of public health interventions in developing countries. However, randomized designs may be better utilized with education programs in which geographically organized public schools offer relatively comparable groups for analysis and where randomized assignment of students and scholarship may occur. A blend of public and private clinics offering services of vastly divergent quality and scope to persons with disease and disabilities poses greater methodological challenges for randomized design.

CHAPTER FIVE

Research and Other Actions to Promote Impact Assessment

The Bill and Melinda Gates Foundation, the World Health Organization, and, increasingly, other global funding organizations such as the World Bank, are vigorously improving the designs of program evaluations to maximize their utility beyond merely serving as an internal management tool to become a global resource for directing evidence-based national and international health policies. For example, the Bill and Melinda Gates Foundation recently sponsored three randomized tuberculosis treatment pilot programs. The World Bank is now funding expansion of the PROGRESA program (see Chapter Four) throughout Mexico and currently is promoting randomized designs to evaluate HIV education programs in Kenya.

Nevertheless, rigorous impact evaluations of large-scale interventions are currently noteworthy exceptions rather than the rule. The Center for Global Development's recent compilation of successful multiyear large interventions to improve global health, where sufficient investment had been made to support impact evaluations, identified only 17 such cases. The authors of the compilation noted that many large-scale interventions have not been evaluated beyond the pilot stage (Levine and What Works Working Group, 2004). A recent in-house review by the World Bank of its billion-dollar-plus portfolio of programs over the past four or five years found that a mere 2 percent of the programs underwent proper evaluation of whether they produced any real impact (Dugger, 2004).

The World Bank has created the Development Impact Evaluation Taskforce to evaluate the long-term impacts of education, health, and public-utility programs. While the World Bank's Operations Evaluation Department has traditionally evaluated whether projects meet their immediate goals, this new taskforce will strategically select projects to measure programs' long-term impacts on poverty. The World Bank is collaborating with the Massachusetts Institute of Technology's Poverty Action Lab to spearhead its large-scale impact evaluations, including randomized trials, of some of its international education programs, including the HIV/AIDS education campaign in Kenyan schools (Kremer and Miguel, 2001). The World Bank's collaborations with external researchers and evaluators represent an important step toward greater openness to outside scrutiny and disclosure. This step also signifies a conceptual shift in program operation from the premise that program sponsors know precisely what needs be done and the only constraint on program success is proper implementation—the "know-do" gap—toward a more fluid experimental paradigm in which continual monitoring and evaluation stimulate perpetual feedback loops of learning and program evolution. This shift, however, creates a potential trade-off between wanting the program to work and knowing why it did or did not work as originally envisioned and subsequently modified. Thoughtful process evaluations can reduce the potential loss of information by providing insights into exactly what the intervention was and how it was modified from its original design over the course of the intervention.

As global health policy becomes increasingly politicized, more organizations, researchers, and local stakeholders feel compelled to further explore the extent to which incremental improvements in program-evaluation rigor produce information of sufficient strength to guide evidence-based, global-health policymaking. In the sections that follow, we outline areas in which additional research or funding policies might promote impact assessments of large-scale interventions. These activities fall into three broad interrelated categories: increasing support for impact evaluations, enhancing resources and technical capacity to conduct program evaluations in developing countries, and improving evaluation methodologies.

Actions to Increase Support for Impact Evaluations

Developing Priorities for Impact Assessments

Rigorous outcome evaluations and impact assessments are invariably costly and time-consuming. The World Bank estimates that a randomized or quasi-experimental impact evaluation can take one to five years to complete, depending on the amount of time it takes the long-term system effects to emerge. The costs can range from $50,000 to $1 million, depending on the complexity and scope of the project, with the typical evaluation costing several hundred thousand dollars (World Bank, 2004b; World Bank Group, 2004). While additional investment in evaluating health interventions is clearly needed, scarce resources and limited evaluative capacity make it particularly important that costly impact assessments be undertaken selectively when they are most likely to produce usable results that will help inform what may work and what may not work. Participants at a 1988 Brookings Institution Symposium on evaluation of complex social interventions cautioned that investments in such evaluations should be undertaken only when (1) there is a theory connecting the interventions, the intermediate surrogate markers, and the expected outcomes (the cause and effect chain), and (2) the interventions are of sufficient scale and intensity to suggest that they will be successful and their results meaningful (Mann, 1998). An evaluation's findings are more likely to be generalizable when there is a theoretical underpinning for an intervention's effectiveness, and an impact evaluation should not be initiated unless the estimate of the intervention's effects will have adequate statistical power to measure outcomes.

A formal framework for deciding when an impact assessment would be appropriate could help funding agencies think more systematically about their evaluative strategies. For example, a formal framework could draw on Bayesian statistical methods as a way to operationalize the pre-existing level of information that is predictive of the intervention's effect and establish tests to determine whether the invention is of sufficient scale for the outcome estimates to have adequate statistical power. The framework could also incorporate considerations to clarify the primary goal of the evaluation—to improve the effectiveness of the particular intervention or to provide information that could be used for future funding decisions.

Using a formal framework as a decisionmaking tool has several advantages. It encourages development of the evaluative strategy in the program design phase. *Ex ante* evaluation designs are likely to be less time- and resource-intensive and more rigorous than post-implementation designs because, for example, control groups, data requirements, and indicators are built in from the outset. Moreover, making decisions on the evaluation strategy during the program design stage may counteract some of the selection biases that are likely to occur with *ex post* selection of comparison groups. A systematic decisionmaking process is also likely to increase understanding of when program-impact evaluation is appropriate, and why evaluations of scaled-up programs are at least as important as pilot demonstrations. When evaluation strategies are determined *ex post,* unsuccessful programs are less likely to be evaluated and, when evaluation does occur, the findings are less likely to be published. Deciding *ex ante* on the evaluative strategy may help to overcome these biases.

Building a Case for Impact Evaluation
The case for impact evaluation rests on two premises: Knowing what works is important for the wise investment of scarce resources for health projects, and knowing the health outcomes and system impacts of successful cost-effective interventions will generate additional investments in health. Funding organizations should view impact evaluations as a way to leverage their investment beyond their financing capabilities. Building evidence and consensus for what works and what does not work avoids wasting resources on interventions for the latter, and it attracts funding for the former.

Funding organizations should see impact evaluations as an "international public good" with benefits extending far beyond the decisions being made within individual organizations (Duflo, 2003). Indeed, the scaling up of the PROGRESA project in Mexico and its expansion to other countries demonstrates the value of rigorous impact evaluations in stimulating additional program investments. More case studies illustrating how impact evaluations have made a difference in funding priorities and program design are needed. They should not only be examples of when impact evaluation has led to decisions to scale up or to replicate programs, but also when it has led to design modifications or to curtailing projects and reallocating funds to more effective interventions.

It is important that a case be developed for evaluations of scaled-up projects. Such evaluations are important because the systemic impacts may be different for a program operating on a larger scale than a program operating on a pilot basis, and intervening events between the pilot stage and the scaled-up intervention may influence results. The challenge is to convince stakeholders of the importance of impact evaluations of scaled-up programs. Stakeholders may believe that such evaluation is unnecessary because findings were already generated from the pilot, and because they have political investment in the project's success and may not want to risk having potentially adverse findings.

It is also important that the case be made for rigorous impact evaluations using randomized designs. Randomized designs raise fewer methodological uncertainties and challenges and are likely to be more influential in the policymaking process for controversial interventions than would quasi-experimental designs that could cause the policy debate to be sidetracked by methodological issues and the soundness of the evaluation results. In this regard, the 2004 World Bank report *Influential Evaluations: Evaluations that Improved Performance and Impacts of Development Programs* provides minimal evidence of real impact evaluation, despite its professed mission to demonstrate the long-term cost-effectiveness of evaluation. The report highlights the limitations of cost-benefit calculations that are based on rather shallow impact evaluations and that fail to capture overall long-term impacts (The World Bank, 2004a).

Encouraging Multidisciplinary Evaluation Designs

Public health has shifted away from a purely medical approach to addressing diseases toward a more fully integrated, multidimensional view of public health programs as inextricably connected to larger social, behavioral, psychological, and economic factors. As public health programs combine their efforts with other disciplines such as education and economic development, the evaluation methods these sectors typically use also must undergo a type of integrative mixing. For example, the development of quality-adjusted life years (QALY) as a standard outcome measure in economic evaluation of health programs results from the integration of economic analysis into health research. While cost-benefit analyses provide a conceptual framework for comparing the value of various program strategies, the ultimate power of these analyses to produce meaningful comparisons relies on the capacity of the impact evaluations to provide comprehensive information on full program effects. While this report has emphasized randomized evaluation designs and statistical techniques for measuring impacts, the strongest impact assessments combine process evaluations and other nonquantitative assessments with quantitative analysis. The process evaluations provide a more thorough understanding of how an intervention was implemented and how it affected the lives of individuals.

Creating Funding Incentives

Funding organizations could create funding incentives, such as the following, to encourage more-rigorous impact evaluations.

- Conditional or staged funding could be used to encourage formative evaluations and prospective evaluation design so that the required data and evaluation metrics are established at the outset of the intervention. Financial support for the data-collection effort could be conditional on the funding recipient strengthening its ongoing data information systems.

- Most projects have a specific amount set aside for funding of program monitoring and evaluation. An "across-the-board" set-aside percentage is unlikely to result in efficient use of evaluation funds. It may provide too much funding for projects requiring only monitoring and insufficient funds when impact evaluation is warranted. An explicit dollar set-aside for an impact evaluation would safeguard the funds for this purpose and assure they are not diverted to ongoing monitoring activities.

- Grants for evaluation activities would be more attractive to government administrators than would loans for this purpose (Duflo, 2003).
- Matching grants or outright grants from international funding organizations could be a way to encourage both nongovernmental organizations and government programs to undertake evaluations.

Actions to Improve Evaluative Capacity

Facilitate Use of Evaluation Methodologies

Researchers are developing standards for reporting of methods, data, and outcomes in order to facilitate interpretation of program evaluations. In March 2004, a team of British statisticians adapted the 2001 Consolidated Standards of Reporting Trials (CONSORT) statement, which includes a checklist of items for standardized reporting of randomized trials in which individuals are randomized to intervention and control groups, such as "cluster" randomized trials typically used by community-wide field trials (Campbell et al., 2004). Such guidelines provide researchers with a general framework for conducting their studies and for presenting their results in a manner conducive to review and further meta-analysis.

Nonrandomized behavioral and public health interventions also suffer from poor reporting and evaluation. The HIV/AIDS Prevention Research Synthesis (PRS) team of the Centers for Disease Control and Prevention (CDC) found significant obstacles to synthesis of study reports due to failure to include critical information, such as intervention timing and dosage and effect-size data (Des Jarlais, 2004). To address these methodological shortcomings, the CDC convened a meeting of medical journal editors in Atlanta in July 2003. The meeting produced the Transparent Reporting of Evaluations with Nonrandomized Designs (TREND) checklist, the nonrandomized version of the CONSORT checklist for randomized designs (Kirkwood, 2004). Space limitations in medical journals may prevent researchers from including full descriptions of theories, prior research results, study designs, and other details in the TREND checklist. Nevertheless, the authors of the TREND checklist hoped that it would encourage researchers to at least consider the items in the checklist when reporting evaluation results and to perhaps publish more-detailed evaluation descriptions on the Internet, and stimulate further dialogue about methodological issues involved in nonrandomized designs. Funding organizations might consider establishing a "warehouse" for evaluations of health interventions and making this information readily available to researchers.

Increase Independent Evaluator Technical Capacity

Rigorous impact evaluations should be conducted by an independent evaluator who has no stake in the outcome of the evaluation. Such evaluations require a high level of specialized expertise in statistical methods. To build program evaluators' expertise, funding agencies should consider collaboratively sponsoring one or more independent multidisciplinary evaluation organizations to serve as resources to other researchers on methodological issues. These organization could

- serve as a resource for researchers on evaluation methodologies and issues
- conduct high-priority randomized impact evaluations that could be used as "best practice" models for evaluation
- provide training and technical assistance for health-services research in developing countries
- maintain an easily accessible repository and/or gateway for evaluations of public-health interventions in developing countries and literature on evaluation methodologies and issues
- foster testing of new evaluation methodologies
- establish partnerships between local projects and researchers
- encourage further standardization of reporting of evaluation findings and of indicators.

Increase Local Evaluation Capacity

Often, actions to develop local evaluative capacity create trade-offs between local capacity-building monitoring and evaluation activities and the traditional focus on accountability and impact and the use of external evaluators. Capacity-building activities are important for project sustainability and for strengthening the local infrastructure to perform evaluations. These activities emphasize participatory monitoring and evaluation activities in which project investigators help organizations to build the internal capacity to evaluate themselves. Local participants' aversion to program evaluation as a time- and resource-draining auditing activity has been overcome when those participants engage with other stakeholders in developing the evaluation design and subsequently buy into the evaluation process. Efficiency and buy-in are further facilitated by the use of a single recordkeeping and data system.

A delicate balance exists between involving local participants in an evaluation process and maintaining the rigor—such as standardized indicators, survey methods, and statistical techniques—needed for credible impact evaluations. Collaborative models that strive for this balance need to be developed and tested so that evaluation activities both build local evaluation capacity and contribute to evidence-based health interventions. Partnerships involving the pairing of experienced evaluators with local evaluators, such as those used by the American International Health Alliance, may provide a model for this activity; however, the success of the model in building evaluation capacity would need to be formally evaluated.

Disseminate Research Findings

Knowing what works and what does not work, with respect to both an entire project and individual components of an intervention, requires having results from both successful and unsuccessful projects being made available. This requires not only stepping up the intensity of efforts for impact evaluation but also widely disseminating findings from the evaluations. Increasing recognition of the importance of building a library of evidence-based medicine in developing countries has been cited in a number of reports, including recent editorials in the *Journal of the American Medical Association* (Buekens et al., 2004) and the *British Medical Journal* (Richards, 2004). The World Bank (World Bank Group, 2004a) has indicated that it will make its impact assessments available online. Increasing the availability of evidence-based evaluations through the Cochrane Collaboration (Richards, 2004) or some other repository offers a way to overcome the bias toward publishing results from only successful interventions.

Actions to Improve Evaluation Methodologies

Although the statistical techniques needed to support impact evaluations have been developed, additional research in several areas would improve impact evaluations. Improvements are needed to increase the quality of impact evaluations and to make them less costly and time-consuming, which in turn would make them more attractive to funding organizations. Some areas that warrant additional attention include the following:

- **Baseline and trend surveys.** Without proper and timely baseline surveys and trend estimates, it is difficult to argue for the effectiveness of any program. Baseline surveys should be an integral part of pre-post surveys and cluster or standard randomized control trials. However, in prospective outcome evaluations based on the "log-frame" approach, they are often omitted. If the baseline survey is not possible for cost or logistical reasons, or if the evaluation is retrospective, a caveat should be included in the evaluation report and explanations should be provided for any point-in-time or trend estimates used for pre-intervention outcome and impact measures.
- **Using a "log-frame" approach where appropriate.** Where controlled trials are not possible, but it is essential to determine the impact of program decisions and investments, the log-frame approach described in Chapter Two could be invaluable. Even retrospective evaluations tracing the successive levels of program impact could credibly connect intermediate outcomes to the observed levels of the final impact of interest. With a proper baseline measurement from sources that are internal or external to

the evaluation, it would then be feasible to illustrate whether a program's effectiveness was as intended.

- **Rapid measurement techniques.** Statistical methodologies for evaluation of health interventions in developing countries are undergoing a rather dynamic period of exploratory experimentation. Researchers are now seeking cost-effective measurement techniques to obtain the quick snapshots of data needed for at least a preliminary sense of trends and real-world program impact. For example, public health researchers have recently adopted the lot quality assurance sampling (LQAS) technique used by the manufacturing industry for quality assurance in order to make swift calculations of high versus low disease prevalence among relatively small population samples. LQAS methodologies work particularly well in areas of high disease prevalence, because the sampling procedures may be terminated mid-sample as soon as the threshold is met; it remains to be seen how successfully LQAS operates in low- and medium-prevalence areas.

- **Surrogate markers.** The assumptions governing the use of surrogate makers need to be evaluated to confirm whether there is a strong link between the surrogate and the desired outcomes.

- **Tracer interventions.** For large integrated health projects, such as PMTCT interventions in which the monitoring and evaluation of all the components of the program may be too cumbersome for local staff, there is an increasing trend toward evaluating the effect of "tracer" interventions. Tracer interventions reflect the trends of the key components of the entire intervention (UNAIDS, 2000). The efficacy of tracer interventions in judging the true effectiveness of an entire program needs to be rigorously analyzed. The advantages and disadvantages of the approach, especially in situations in which the program is a joint TB-HIV intervention, or a joint effort on endemic diseases including malaria, need to be assessed.

- **Contextual measures.** Better indicators are needed to measure environmental features—such as organizational capacity and leadership commitment—which may affect the likelihood of an intervention's success and/or be indirectly affected by the intervention.

- **Nonbiological effects.** Considerably more attention should be given to standardizing indicators to measure the nonbiological effects of health interventions on individuals, their families, and their communities and to developing rapidly assayable survey methods for collecting data on these measures. The cost effectiveness of an intervention may not be correctly estimated unless these effects are taken into account.

- **Strengthening surveillance.** Further strengthening of ongoing data-collection systems and standardization of measures should reduce the costs of data collection for evaluations and facilitate cross-site comparisons.

Increasing support for impact evaluations, enhancing evaluative capacity, and improving evaluation methodologies should help to close the gap between "best practices" in program evaluation and evaluative strategies being used in actual practice. There is general agreement that rigorous program evaluation of interventions in various resource-limited settings is needed to know which interventions will work most effectively and to spend scarce resources wisely. What is not clear, however, is the extent to which incremental improvements in program-evaluation rigor produce information of sufficient strength to guide evidence-based, global-health policymaking. Current levels of evaluation are clearly insufficient. However, the scope of future evaluations must be carefully calibrated to match the scope of the intervention, and techniques must be properly selected to match the level of precision required by the type of information sought. Researchers must be up front about the limitations of their methods to capture a range of effects and must explore new methods of capturing larger effects, which may require more qualitative reasoning, because higher statistical rigor may exclude important larger insights. Indeed, as the evidence-based, public-health movement presses for more rigorous evaluation, these evaluations themselves must be continuously scrutinized for appropriateness.

HIV/AIDS Data Sources

Data Source	Description	Date	Data Collection and Dissemination
Demographic Health Survey (DHS+)	Principal funding from USAID, with some DHS surveys co-funded by UNFPA, World Bank, WHO, and others. Started as a successor to the World Fertility Study (WFS) and Contraceptive Prevalence Survey (CPS), DHS is administered by Macro Evaluation as part of the MEASURE/DHS+ project (Boerma and Sommerfelt, 1993). DHS surveys are nationally representative household surveys with large sample sizes of 5,000 to 30,000 households typically. DHS surveys provide data for a wide range of monitoring and impact evaluation indicators in the areas of population, health, and nutrition. Data are now available for 51 countries. Additional modules have been added over time (e.g., HIV/AIDS indicators were added in the early 1990s).	1984–present	Repeat surveys are conducted at three- and five-year intervals. Countries administering the DHS surveys are responsible for absorbing a portion of the costs, which may impact the countries' ability to conduct repeat surveys. Data are typically available 8 to 12 months after survey completion.
Reproductive Health Survey (RHS)	Funded by USAID, and administered by CDC, these surveys measure a wide variety of health and demographic indicators such as fertility, contraceptive use, infant and child mortality, child health, maternal morbidity and mortality, and knowledge and attitudes about HIV/AIDS and sexually transmitted infections.	1975–present	

Data Source	Description	Date	Data Collection and Dissemination
Behavioral Surveillance Survey (BSS)	Funded by USAID and administered by Family Health International (FHI) through its IMPACT project, the BSS tracks HIV-risk populations over time and is especially useful in providing information for subpopulations who may be difficult to reach through the DHS+ survey, particularly high-risk groups. The BSS has been implemented in more than 33 countries to date (Family Health International, 2002).	1997– present	Estimated time required for conducting a BSS from the start of the protocol development until dissemination ranges from 43 to 49 weeks, depending on the country. Surveys are conducted on an annual basis, but the countries that choose to participate vary from year to year (Family Health International, 2002).
UNAIDS General Population Survey	Funded by UNAIDS, this survey was designed to provide information on topics explicitly related to HIV/AIDS, including background, knowledge of HIV/AIDS, sexual behavior, marriage and partnerships, exposure to HIV/AIDS interventions, attitudes toward people with HIV/AIDS, and other such topics.	1996– present	
UNAIDS/WHO Epidemiological Fact Sheets	Funded by UNAIDS and WHO, the fact sheets collate the most recent country-specific data on HIV/AIDS prevalence and incidence and information on HIV/AIDS behaviors.	1996– present	Data are collected on an annual basis from national AIDS programs, national institutions, and international experts and institutions. New fact sheets are disseminated each year. UNAIDS and WHO do not collect the primary data. Information for every indicator is not available for all countries. The time from data collection to dissemination varies by country (UNAIDS, WHO, and UNICEF, 2002).

Data Source	Description	Date	Data Collection and Dissemination
Multiple Indicator Cluster Survey (MICS)	UNICEF and a number of partners first developed the MICS in 1992 to monitor the goals of the World Summit for Children in 1990. By 1996, 60 countries completed this mid-decade assessment, and 40 others had incorporated MICS modules into existing surveys. Drawing from lessons learned from the mid-decade assessment, the end-of-decade assessment was developed specifically to obtain the data for 63 of the 75 end-decade indicators. Indicators included in the survey are nutrition, health and education, birth registration, family environment, child work, and knowledge of HIV/AIDS (UNICEF, no date).	1992– present	Data are collected on an annual basis. However, different indicators are collected within varying time frames. For example, underweight prevalence is measured every three years, while the literacy rate is measured every five years. Data collection also varies by country depending on availability (UNICEF, 1999).
World Development Indicators	Funded by The World Bank, these indicators are a compilation of primary and secondary data organized into six sections: World View, People, Environment, Economy, States and Markets, and Global Links. The People section collects data on health expenditures, services, and use; access to health services; reproductive health; risk factors and future challenges; and mortality, among other indicators.	1997– present	The World Bank is not a primary data collection agency other than for living-standards surveys and data on foreign debt. Given that The World Bank collects data from a variety of sources, differences in the methods and conventions used by the primary data collectors may give rise to significant discrepancies over time both among and within countries. Delays in reporting data and the use of old surveys as the base for current estimates may sometimes compromise the quality of national data. In an effort to improve data collection efforts in developing countries, The World Bank funds and participates in technical assistance efforts.

Data Source	Description	Date	Data Collection and Dissemination
World Development Indicators

(continued) | | | Data are reported on an annual basis; updated data for each country are not always available. The time from data collection to dissemination varies by country (The World Bank, 1998). |

Bibliography

Acevado, W., A. Afani, M. Ayala et al., "Primary Resistance in HIV Chilean Patients," program and abstracts of the *XV International AIDS Conference*, Bangkok, July 11–16, 2004.

Adatu, F., R. Odeke, M. Mugenyi et al., "Implementation of the DOTS Strategy for Tuberculosis Control in Rural Kiboga District, Uganda, Offering Patients the Option of Treatment Supervision in the Community, 1998–1999," *International Journal of Tuberculosis and Lung Disease,* Vol. 7, No. 9, Supplement 1, 2003 pp. S63–S71.

Ainsworth, M., "Assessing M&E of National HIV/AIDS Programs: Findings from Four Developing Countries," program and abstracts of the XV International AIDS Conference, Bangkok, July 11–16, 2004.

Andrews, G. V., "Nobody Here Wants to Admit They Have AIDS . . . They All Have TB: Evaluation of a HIV/AIDS Home-Based Care Programme for Ex-miners, South Africa," program and abstracts of the XV International AIDS Conference, Bangkok, Thailand, July 11–16, 2004.

Atabaki, N., "The World Bank Is Finally Embracing Science," *The Lancet,* Vol. 364, August 27, 2004 pp. 731–732.

Badri, M., D. Wilson, and R. Wood, "Effect of Highly Active Antiretroviral Therapy on Incidence of Tuberculosis in South Africa: A Cohort Study," *The Lancet,* Vol. 359, 2002, pp. 2059–2064.

Bamberger, M., *Influential Evaluations: Evaluations that Improved Performance and Impacts of Development Programs*, Washington, D.C.: The World Bank, 2004.

Barreto, M. L., "Design of the Brazilian BCG-REVAC Trial Against Tuberculosis: A Large Simple Randomized Community Trial to Evaluate the Impact on Tuberculosis of BCG Revaccination at School Age," *Controlled Clinical Trials*, Vol. 23, October 2002, pp. 540–553.

Bennett, S., D. Braunholtz, S. Chinn et al., "Cluster Randomized Trials: Methodological and Ethical Considerations," UK: *MRC Clinical Trial Series*, November 2002.

Beyer, J. A., "The Role of the World Bank in International Health: Renewed Commitment and Partnership," *Social Science and Medicine*, Vol. 50, pp. 169–176.

Bobonis, G. J., E. Miguel, and C. Puri Sharma, "Iron Deficiency Anemia and School Participation," *Poverty Action Lab Paper No. 7*, Cambridge, Mass: Massachusetts Institute of Technology, 2004.

Boerma, J. T., and A. E. Sommerfelt, "Demographic and Health Surveys (DHS): Contributions and Limitations," *Health Statistics Quarterly*, Vol. 46, No. 4, 1993, pp. 222–226.

Breman, J. G., M. S. Alilio, and A. Mills, "Conquering the Intolerable Burden of Malaria: What's New, What's Needed: A Summary," *The American Journal of Tropical Medicine and Hygiene*, Vol. 71, Supplement 2, August 2004, pp. 1–15.

Brody, B. A., "Ethical Issues in Clinical Trials in Developing Countries," *Statistics in Medicine*, Vol. 21, October 2002, pp. 2853–2858.

Bryce, J., "The Multi-Country Evaluation of the Integrated Management of Childhood Illness Strategy: Lessons for the Evaluation of Public Health Interventions," *Public Health Matters*, Vol. 94, No. 3, March 2004, pp. 406-415.

Buekens, P., G. Keusch, J. Belizan, and Z. Ahmed Bhutta, "Evidence-Based Global Health," *Journal of the American Medical Association*, Vol. 291, No. 21, June 2, 2004, pp. 2639–2641.

Butt, T., R. N. Ahmad, S. Y. Kazmi et al. "Rapid Diagnosis of Pulmonary Tuberculosis by Mycobacteriophage Assay," *International Journal of Tuberculosis and Lung Disease*, Vol. 8, No. 7, 2004, pp. 889–890.

Campbell, M. K., D. R. Elbourne, and D. G. Altman, "CONSORT Statement: Extension to Cluster Randomised Trials," *British Journal of Medicine*, Vol. 328, March 20, 2004, pp. 702–708.

Chun, T., G. Zellman, B. M. Stecher, and E. Giddens, *An Evaluation Strategy Developed by RAND for the Broad Foundation*, Santa Monica, Calif.: RAND Corporation, DRU-2612-EDU, 2001.

Clark, M., and R. Sartorius, "Monitoring and Evaluation: Some Tools, Methods, and Approaches," Washington, D.C.: *The World Bank*, 2004.

Clemens, J., "Evaluating New Vaccines for Developing Countries: Efficacy or Effectiveness?" *Journal of the American Medical Association*, Vol. 275, No. 5, February 7, 1996, pp. 390–397.

Cohen, S. A., "Beyond Slogans: Lessons from Uganda's Experience with ABC and HIV/AIDS," *The Guttmacher Report on Public Policy*, December 2003, pp. 1–3.

Collins, C. D., "The Relationship Between Disease Control Strategies and Health System Development: The Case of TB," *Health Policy*, Vol. 62, November 2002, pp. 141–160.

Cowan, F. M., L. F. Langhaug, G. P. Mashungupa et al., "School-Based HIV Prevention in Zimbabwe: Feasibility and Acceptability of Evaluation Trials Using Biological Outcomes," *AIDS*, Vol. 16, 2002, pp. 1673–1678.

Council for International Organizations of Medical Sciences (CIOMS), *International Ethical Guidelines for Biomedical Research Involving Human Subjects*, Geneva, Switzerland: *CIOMS*, 2002.

Davey, S., *State of the World's Vaccines and Immunization*, Geneva, Switzerland: The World Health Organization, 2002.

Davies P.D.O., "The Role of DOTS in Tuberculosis Treatment and Control," *American Journal of Respiratory Medicine*, Vol. 2, No. 3, 2003, pp. 203–209.

Dayan, G., "Cost-Effectiveness of Three Different Vaccination Strategies Against Measles in Zambian Children," *Vaccine*, Vol. 22, January 2004, pp. 475–484.

De Cock, K. M., "Prevention of Mother-to-Child HIV Transmission in Resource-Poor Countries: Translated Research into Policy and Practice," *Journal of the American Medical Association*, Vol. 283, No. 9, March 1, 2000, pp. 1175–1182.

Des Jarlais, D. C., "Issues in HIV Prevention for Injecting Drug Users (IDUs) in Developing/Transitional Countries: Results from the WHO

Phase II Drug Injection Study," Bangkok, Thailand: XV International AIDS Conference, July 11–16, 2004.

Donner, A., G. Giaggio, and J. Villar, "Meta-analysis of Cluster Randomized Trials: Power Considerations," *Evaluation and the Health Professions*, Vol. 26, No. 3, September 2003, pp. 340–351.

Donner, A., and N. Klar, eds., "Cluster Randomization Trials," *Statistical Methods in Medical Research*, Vol. 9, 2002, pp. 79–179.

___. "Issues in the Meta-Analysis of Cluster Randomized Trials," *Statistics in Medicine*, Vol. 21, October 2002, pp. 2971–2980.

Dow, W. H., J. Holmes, T. Philipson, and X. Sala-i-Martin, *Disease Complementarities and the Evaluation of Public Health Interventions*, Cambridge, Mass.: National Bureau of Economic Research, 1995.

Duflo, E., "Scaling-up Evaluation," paper prepared for *ABCDE* in Bangalore, India, May 13, 2003.

Dugger, C., "World Bank Challenged: Are the Poor Really Helped?" *The New York Times*, July 28, 2004.

Dyer, C., "The Science of Social Diseases," *Science*, Vol. 307, 2005, p. 181.

Dyer, C. B., G. Williams, M. A. Espinal, and M. C. Raviglione, "Erasing the World's Slow Stain: Strategies to Beat Multidrug-Resistant Tuberculosis," *Science*, Vol. 295, 2002, pp. 2042–2046.

Erulkar, A. S., L.I.A. Ettyang, C. Onoka et al., "Behavior Change Evaluation of a Culturally Consistent Reproductive Health Program for Young Kenyans," *International Family Planning Perspectives*, Vol. 30, No. 2, 2004, pp. 58–67.

Family Health International, "FHI Evaluating Program Effectiveness Guide" (www.fhi.org/en/HIVAIDS/pub/fact/evalprog.htm, accessed January 25, 2005).

Family Health International, "Implementing Behavioral Surveillance Surveys: Guidance to the Field," PowerPoint presentation, June 2002.

Family Health International (AIDSCAP Project), "Module 3: A Framework for Incorporating Evaluation into Project Design," Arlington, Va.: Family Health International, 1997.

Floyd, K., "Existing Evidence on the Cost-Effectiveness of TB and HIV/AIDS Interventions in Developing Countries: A Review,"

PowerPoint presentation, DCPP Economics Workshop, Bethesda, Md., November 5–7, 2002.

Gallant, M., and E. Maticka-Tyndale, "School-Based HIV Prevention Programmes for African Youth," *Social Science & Medicine*, Vol. 58, No. 7, 2004, pp. 1337–1351.

Garfield, R., "Malaria Control in Nicaragua: Social and Political Influences on Disease Transmission and Control Activities," *The Lancet*, Vol. 354, July 31, 1999, pp. 414–418.

Glasgow, R. E., E. Lichtenstein, and A. Marcus, "Why Don't We See More Translation of Health Promotion Research to Practice? Rethinking the Efficacy-to-Effectiveness Transition," *Public Health Matters*, Vol. 93, No. 8, pp. 1261–1267.

Glasgow, R. E., T. M. Vogt, and S. M. Boles, "Evaluating the Public Health Impact of Health Promotion Interventions: The RE-AIM Framework," *American Journal of Public Health*, Vol. 89, No. 9, pp. 1322–1327.

Gonzalez-Block, M., and A. Mills, "Assessing Capacity for Health Policy and Systems Research in Low- and Middle-Income Countries," *Health Research Policy and Systems*, Vol. 1, No. 1, November 2004.

Grantham, L. N., P. McGluwa, B. A. Biggar et al., "Data Management in a Resource Limited Setting," program and abstracts of the XV International AIDS Conference, Bangkok, Thailand, July 11–16, 2004.

Grassly, N. C. et al. "Uncertainty in Estimates of HIV/AIDS: The Estimation and Application of Plausibility Bounds," *Sexually Transmitted Infections*, Vol. 80, No. 4, Supplement 1, 2004, pp. i31–i38.

Grasso, P. G., S. W. Wasty, and R. V. Weaving, *World Bank Operations Evaluation Development: The First 30 Years*, Washington, D.C.: The World Bank, 2003.

Greenwood, B., "Between Hope and Hard Place," *Nature*, Vol. 430, August 19, 2004, pp. 926–927.

Gupta, P., C. Pant, K. Peteres, and R. Vandendries, *What Have We Learned? Some Preliminary Lessons from OED's Country Assistance Evaluations*, Washington, D.C.: The World Bank, 2004.

Gupta, R., J. Y. Kim, M. A. Espinal, J. M. Caudron, B. Pecoul, P. E. Farmer, and M. C. Raviglione, "Public Health: Responding to Market

Failures in Tuberculosis Control," *Science,* Vol. 293, 2001, pp. 1049–1051.

Gupte, M. D., B. N. Murthy, K. Mahmood, S. Meeralakshmi, B. Nagaraju, and R. Prabhakaran, "Application of Lot Quality Assurance Sampling for Leprosy Elimination Monitoring—Examination of Some Critical Factors," *International Journal of Epidemiology*, Vol. 33, August 28, 2003, pp. 344–348.

Harms, G., S. Theuring, A. Mayer et al., "Cost Evaluation of PMTCT Programmes," program and abstracts of the XV International AIDS Conference, Bangkok, Thailand, July 11–16, 2004.

Hayes, R. J., N.D.E. Alexander, S. Bennett, and S. N. Cousens, "Design and Analysis Issues in Cluster-Randomized Trials of Interventions Against Infectious Disease," *Statistical Methods in Medical Research*, Vol. 9, April 2000, pp. 95–116.

Heinrich, C. J., and J. B. Wenger, "The Economic Contributions of James J. Heckman and Daniel McFadden," *Review of Political Economy*, Vol. 14, No. 1, January 2002, p. 69.

Hill, P. S., "The Rhetoric of Sector-wide Approaches for Health Development," *Social Science and Medicine*, Vol. 54, 2002, pp. 1725–1737.

Hohmann, A., and M. Katherine Shear, "Community-Based Intervention Research: Coping with the 'Noise' of Real Life in Study Design," *American Journal of Psychiatry*, Vol. 159, No. 2, February 2002, pp. 201–207.

Hoshaw-Woodard, S., *Description and Comparison of the Methods of Cluster Sampling and Lot Quality Assurance Sampling to Assess Immunization Coverage*, Geneva: World Health Organization, 2001.

Hosseinipour, M. C., P. N. Kazembe, I. M. Sanne, and C. M. van der Horst, "Challenges in Delivering Antiretroviral Treatment in Resource Poor Countries," *AIDS*, Vol. 16, Supplement 4, pp. 2002, S177–S187.

Hudson, C. P., "Community-Based Trials of Sexually Transmitted Disease Treatment: Repercussions for Epidemiology and HIV Prevention," *Bulletin of the World Health Organization*, Vol. 79, No. 7, 2001, pp. 48–58.

Isaakidis, P., and J.P.A. Ioannidis, "Evaluation of Cluster Randomized Controlled Trials in Sub-Saharan Africa," *American Journal of Epidemiology*, Vol. 158, No. 9, November 1, 2003, pp. 921–926.

Janz, N. K., M. A. Zimmerman, P. A. Wren et al., "Evaluation of 37 AIDS Prevention Projects: Successful Approaches and Barriers to Program Effectiveness," *Health Education Quarterly*, Vol. 123, No. 1, 1996, pp. 80–97.

Jaratsist, S., "Evaluation of AIDS Case Reporting System," program and abstracts of the XV International AIDS Conference, Bangkok, Thailand, July 11–16, 2004.

Johnston, T., and S. Stout, *Investing in Health: Development Effectiveness in the Health, Nutrition, and Population Sector*, Washington, D.C.: The World Bank, 1999.

Judd, J., "Setting Standards in the Evaluation of Community-Based Health Promotion Programmes—A Unifying Approach," *Health Promotion International*, Vol. 16, No. 4, 2001, pp. 367–379.

Kakande, C., and S. D. Bunyole, "HIV/AIDs Project Evaluation," program and abstracts of the XV International AIDS Conference, Bangkok, Thailand, July 11–16, 2004.

Kamali, A., "Syndromic Management of Sexually Transmitted Infections and Behavior Change Interventions on Transmission of HIV-1 in Rural Uganda: A Community Randomized Trial," *The Lancet*, Vol. 361, February 22, 2004, pp. 645–652.

Kapp, C., "Hazard or Help?" *The Lancet*, Vol. 364, September 25, 2004, pp. 1113–1114.

Kassa, E., R. de Wit, F. Tobias et al., "Evaluation of the WHO Staging System for HIV Infection and Disease in Ethiopia: Association Between Clinical Stages and Laboratory Markers," *AIDS*, Vol. 13, No. 3, 1999, pp. 381–389.

Kazeonny, B., T. Khorosheva, T. Aptekar et al., "Evaluation of a Directly Observed Therapy Short-Course Strategy for Treating Tuberculosis—Orel Oblast, Russian Federation, 1999–2000," *Centers for Disease Control and Prevention Weekly*, Vol. 50, No. 11, March 23, 2001, pp. 204–206.

Kegeles, S. M., G. M. Rebchook, S. Tebbetts et al., "Perspectives on Barriers and Facilitators to Community-Based Organizations (CBOs) Evaluation of Their HIV Prevention Efforts," program and abstracts of the XV International AIDS Conference, Bangkok, Thailand, July 11–16, 2004.

Kent, D. M., "Suitable Monitoring Approaches to Antiretroviral Therapy in Resource-Poor Settings: Setting the Research Agenda," *Clinical Infectious Diseases,* Vol. 37, Supplement 1, July 1, 2003, pp. S13–S24.

___. "Clinical Trials in Sub-Saharan Africa and Established Standards of Care: A Systematic Review of HIV, Tuberculosis, and Malaria Trials," *Journal of the American Medical Association,* Vol. 292, No. 2, July 14, 2004, pp. 237–243.

Kent, D., D. McGrath, J.P.A. Ioannidis et al., "Suitable Monitoring Approaches to Antiretroviral Therapy in Resource-Poor Settings: Setting the Research Agenda," *Clinical Infectious Diseases,* Vol. 37, Supplement 1, 2003, pp. S13–S24.

Kim, J. Y., "PIH Testimony to Senate Foreign Relations Committee," *Senate Foreign Relations Sub-Committee on African Affairs,* (http://www.phrusa.org/campaigns/aids/news0214.html, accessed February 14, 2002).

Kirkwood, B., "Making Public Health Interventions More Evidence Based: TREND Statement for Non-Randomized Designs Will Make a Difference," *British Journal of Medicine,* Vol. 328, April 24, 2004, pp. 966–967.

Kremer, M., and E. Miguel, "Worms: Education and Health Externalities in Kenya," *Poverty Action Lab,* National Bureau of Economic Research (NBER) Working Paper W8481, 2001.

Levine, R., and the What Works Working Group with Molly Kinder, *Millions Saved: Proven Successes in Global Health*, Washington, D.C.: Center for Global Development, 2004.

Lewin, S., J. Dick, M. Zwarenstein, and C. J. Lombard, "Staff Training and Ambulatory Tuberculosis Treatment Outcomes: A Cluster Randomized Controlled Trial in South Africa," *Bulletin of the World Health Organization,* Vol. 83, No. 4, April 2005, pp. 250–259.

Lindblade, K., et al., "Sustainability of Reductions in Malaria Transmission and Infant Mortality in Western Kenya With Use of Insecticide-Treated Bednets: 4 to 6 Years of Follow-up," *Journal of the American Medical Association,* Vol. 291, No. 21, June 2, 2004, pp. 2571–2580.

Maiorana, A., S. Kegeles, C. Sandoval et al., "Process Evaluation for a Behavioral Intervention Outcome Trial in Peru," program and abstracts of the XV International AIDS Conference, Bangkok, Thailand, July 11–16, 2004.

Mann, T. E., "Learning What Works: Evaluating Complex Social Interventions," Washington, D.C.: The Brookings Institution, March 1, 1998 (http://www.brookings.edu/views/articles/mann/1998rf0301.htm, accessed July 2005).

Mantell, J. E., A. T. DiVittis, and M. I. Auerbach, *Evaluating HIV Prevention Interventions*, New York: Plenum Press, 1997.

MAP (Monitoring the AIDS Pandemic), "The Status and Trends of The HIV/AIDS Epidemics In the World," Barcelona Map Symposium, 2002.

McPherson, S., F. Samuels, P. Chikukwa et al., "Getting It Right: Designing an Evaluation of an INGO-Led HIV/AIDS Prevention Programme in Resource Poor Settings," program and abstracts of the XV International AIDS Conference, Bangkok, Thailand, July 11–16, 2004.

Mehret, M., T. E. Mertens, M. Carael et al., "Baseline for the Evaluation of an AIDS Programme Using Prevention Indicators: A Case Study in Ethiopia," *Bulletin of the World Health Organization*, Vol. 74, No. 5, 1996, pp. 509–516.

Mertens, T. E., and M. Carael, "Evaluation of HIV/STD Prevention, Care and Support: An Update on WHO's Approaches," *AIDS Education & Prevention*, Vol. 9, No. 2, 1997, pp. 133–145.

Miti, S., V. Mfungwe, P. Reijer et al., "Integration of Tuberculosis Treatment in a Community-Based Home Care Programme for Persons Living with HIV/AIDS in Ndola, Zambia," *International Journal of Tuberculosis and Lung Disease*, Vol. 7, No. 9, Supplement 1, 2003, pp. S92–S98.

Murray, C.J.L., "Validity of Reported Vaccination Coverage in 45 Countries," in C.J.L. Murray and D. B. Evans, eds., *Health Systems Performance Assessment*, Geneva, Switzerland: World Health Organization, 2003, pp. 265–271.

____. "Towards Evidence-based Public Health," in C.J.L. Murray and D. B. Evans, eds., *Health Systems Performance Assessment*, Geneva: World Health Organization, 2003, pp. 715–725.

Myatt, M., H. Limburg, D. Minassian, and D. Katyola, "Field Trial of Applicability of Lot Quality Assurance Sampling Survey Method for Rapid Assessment of Prevalence of Active Trachoma," *Bulletin of the World Health Organization*, Vol. 81, December 2003, pp. 877–885.

Nateniyom, S., S. X. Hittimanee, N. Ngamtrairai et al., "Implementation of the DOTS Strategy in Prisons at Provincial Level, Thailand," *International Journal of Tuberculosis and Lung Disease*, Vol. 8, No. 7, 2003, pp. 848–854.

Ngamvithayapong, J., W. Uthaivoravit, H. Yanai, P. Akarasewi, and P. Sawanpanyalert, "Adherence to Tuberculosis Preventive Therapy Among HIV-Infected Persons in Chiang Rai, Thailand," *AIDS*, Vol. 11, No. 1, January 11, 1997, pp. 107–112.

Norval, P. Y., K. K. San, T. Bakhim, D. N. Rith, D. I. Ahn, and L. Blanc, "DOTS in Cambodia: Directly Observed Treatment with Short-Course Chemotherapy," *The International Journal of Tuberculosis and Lung Disease*, January 1998, pp. 44–51.

Nuffield Council on Bioethics, *The Ethics of Research Related to Health Care in Developing Countries*, London, UK: Nuffield Council on Bioethics, 2002.

O'Connell, A. A., and D. B. McCoach, "Applications of Hierarchical Linear Models for Evaluation of Health Interventions: Demystifying the Methods and Interpretations of Multilevel Models," *Evaluation & the Health Professions*, Vol. 27, No. 2, June 2004, pp. 119–151.

Office of Communicable Disease Control Region 10, Chiang Mai, Department of Communicable Disease Control, Ministry of Public Health, Thailand, WHO-Thailand, *Isoniazid Preventive Therapy (IPT) for People with HIV in the Upper North of Thailand*, Bangkok, Thailand: Ministry of Public Health, December 2000.

Ohno-Machado, L., "Decision Trees and Fuzzy Logic: A Comparison of Models for the Selection of Measles Vaccination Strategies in Brazil," *Proc AMIA Symposium*, 2000, pp. 625–629.

Orroth, K. K., E. L. Korenromp, R. G. While, J. Changalucha, S. J. de Vlas, R. H. Gray, P. Hughtes, A. Kamali, A. Ojwiya, D. Serwadda, M. J. Wawer, R. J. Hayes, and H. Grosskurth, "Comparison of STD Prevalences in the Mwanza, Rakai, and Masaka Trial Populations: The Role of Selection Bias and Diagnostic Errors," *Sexually Transmitted Infections*, Vol. 79, 2003, pp. 98–105.

Paul, Y., "Herd Immunity and Herd Protection," *Vaccine*, Vol. 22, July 2004, pp. 301–302.

Pope, D. S., and R. E. Chaisson, "TB Treatment: As Simple as DOT," *International Journal of Tuberculosis and Lung Disease*, Vol. 7, No. 7, 2003, pp. 611–615.

Rhodes, S. D., and R. Arceo, "Developing and Testing Measures Predictive of Hepatitis A Vaccination in a Sample of Men Who Have Sex with Men," *Health Education Research*, Vol. 19, No. 3, June 1, 2004, pp. 272–283.

Richards, T., "Poor Countries Lack Relevent Health Information, Says Cochrane Editorial," *British Medical Journal*, 2004.

Rivera, J. A., "Impact of the Mexican Program for Education, Health, and Nutrition (Progresa) on Rates of Growth and Anemia in Infants and Young Children: A Randomized Effectiveness Study," *Journal of the American Medical Association*, Vol. 291, No. 21, June 2, 2004, pp. 2563–2570.

Rossi, P. H., H. E. Freeman, and M. W. Lipsey, *Evaluation: A Systematic Approach*, 6th ed., London: Sage Publications, 1999.

Rotheram-Borus, M. J., "Six-Year Intervention Outcomes for Adolescent Children of Parents with the Human Immunodeficiency Virus," *Archives of Pediatric & Adolescent Medicine*, Vol. 158, August 2004, pp. 742–748.

Royall, J., "Tying-up Lions: Multilateral Initiative on Malaria Communications: the First Chapter of a Malaria Research Network in Africa," *American Journal of Tropical Medicine and Hygiene*, Vol. 71, No. 2, Supplement 2, August 2004, pp. 259–267.

Ruohonen, R. P., T. M. Goloubeva, L. Trnka et al. "Implementation of the DOTS Strategy for Tuberculosis in the Leningrad Region, Russian Federation (1998–1999)," *International Journal of Tuberculosis and Lung Disease*, Vol. 6, No. 3, 2002, pp. 192–197.

Sallet, J., M. Duckworth, G. Mateta et al., "Preparing Managers at District Level to Monitor HIV/AIDS Services," program and abstracts of the *XV International AIDS Conference*, Bangkok, Thailand, July 11–16, 2004.

Scotland, G., E. R. van Teijlingen, M. van der Pol et al., "A Review of Studies Assessing the Costs and Consequences of Interventions to Reduce Mother-to-Child HIV Transmission in Sub-Saharan Africa," *AIDS*, Vol. 17, 2003, pp. 1045–1052.

Sethi, A. K., J. E. Gallant, S. J. Gange et al., "Impact of Current Illicit Drug Use on the Relative Time from Viral Suppression to Rebound with Clinically Significant Drug Resistance Among Patients Receiving Highly Active Antiretroviral Therapy," program and abstracts of the XV International AIDS Conference, Bangkok, Thailand, July 11–16, 2004.

Shantha, S., M. Ramachandran, S. Nataraj et al., "Evaluation of Hospital VCT Services, India," program and abstracts of the XV International AIDS Conference, Bangkok, Thailand, July 11–16, 2004.

Shepard, D. S., "Cost-Effectiveness of the Expanded Programme on Immunization in the Ivory Coast: A Preliminary Assessment," *Social Science Medicine*, Vol. 22, No. 3, 1986, pp. 369–377.

Singh, A. A., D. Parasher, G. S. Shekavat et al., "Effectiveness of Urban Community Volunteers in Directly Observed Treatment of Tuberculosis Patients: A Field Report from Haryana, North India," *International Journal of Tuberculosis and Lung Disease*, Vol. 8, No. 6, 2004, pp. 800–802.

Snow, R. W., "Pediatric Mortality in Africa: Plasmodium Falciparum Malaria as a Cause or Risk?" *American Journal of Tropical Medicine and Hygiene*, Vol. 71, Supplement 2, August 2004, pp. 16–24.

Todd, J., L. Carpenter, Xianbin Li, J. Nakiyingi, R. Gray, and R. Hayes, "The Effects of Alternative Study Designs on the Power of Community Randomized Trials: Evidence from Three Studies of Human Immunodeficiency Virus Prevention in East Africa," *International Journal of Epidemiology*, Vol. 32, No. 5, 2003, pp. 755–762.

Trostle, J., "How Do Researchers Influence Decision-makers? Case Studies of Mexican Politics," *Health Policy and Planning*, Vol. 14, No. 2, June 1999, pp. 103–114.

UN Millennium Project, *Interim Report of Task Force 5 Working Group on HIV/AIDS*, New York, N.Y.: UN Millennium Project, 2004.

UN Roll Back Malaria, "2001–2010 United Nations Decade to Roll Back Malaria: Monitoring and Evaluation" 2005 (http://www.rbm.who.int/cmc_upload/0/000/015/362/RBM Infosheet_11.htm, accessed January 2005).

UNAIDS, "National AIDS Programmes: A Guide to Monitoring and Evaluation," 2000 (http://www.unaids.org/publications/documents/

epidemiology/surveillance/JC427-Mon&Ev-Full-E.pdf, accessed September 2004).

UNAIDS, WHO, and UNICEF, "Epidemiological Fact Sheets by Country," 2002, (http://www.who.int/emc-hiv/fact_sheets/All_ countries. html, accessed August 2005).

United Nations Children's Fund (UNICEF), "UNICEF Statistics: End-of-Decade Assessment Multiple Indicator Cluster Survey," no date (http://www. childinfo.org/MICS2/Gj99306m.htm, accessed September 2004).

___. "UNICEF Executive Directive: End-Decade Assessment—Indicators for Assessing Progress Globally," PowerPoint presentation, April 23, 1999.

USAID, "Thirty Years of USAID Efforts in Population and Health Data Collection: HIV/AIDS," PowerPoint briefing, Washington D.C., June 3, 2002.

USAID, UNAIDS, UNICEF, WHO, and CDC, *HIV/AIDS Survey Indicator Database*, 2005 (http://www.measuredhs.com/hivdata/start. cfm, accessed January 2005).

Vaccine Assessment and Monitoring Team, Department of Immunization, Vaccines, and Biologicals, World Health Organization, *Vaccine-Preventable Diseases: Monitoring System 2004 Global Summary*, Geneva, Switzerland: WHO, November 2004.

Van der Horst, C., "Low-Cost Technologies for Diagnosing and Monitoring HIV-Infected Patients in Resource-Poor Settings," MedScape CME for XIV International AIDS Conference, July 7–12, 2002 (http://www.medscape.com/viewprogram/1986__index; last accessed August 2005).

Vermund, S. H., and W. G. Powderly, "Developing a HIV/AIDS Therapeutic Research Agenda for Resource-limited Countries: A Consensus Statement," *Clinical Infectious Diseases*, Vol. 37, Supplement 1, 2003, pp. S4–S12.

Victoria, C. G., "Evidence-Based Public Health: Moving Beyond Clinical Trials," *Public Health Matters*, Vol. 94, No. 3, March 2004, pp. 400–405.

Volberding, P. A., "Opportunities and Options for Treatment Research in Resource-Constrained Settings," *Clinical Infectious Diseases*, Vol. 37, Supplement 1, 2003, pp. S1–S3.

Walley, J. D., M. A. Khan, J. N. Newell, and M. H. Khan, "Effectiveness of the Direct Observation Component of DOTS for Tuberculosis: A Randomised Controlled Trial in Pakistan," *Lancet*, March 3, 2001, pp. 664–669.

Wilson, T. E., "Changes in Sexual Behavior Among HIV-Infected Women After Initiation of HAART," *American Journal of Public Health*, Vol. 94, No. 7, July 2004, pp. 1141–1147.

The Working Group on Priority Setting, Council on Health Research for Development, "Priority Setting for Health Research: Lessons from Developing Countries," *Health Policy and Planning*, Vol. 15, No. 2, 2002, pp. 130–136.

The World Bank, *Influential Evaluations: Evaluations that Improved Performance and Impacts of Development Programs*, Washington, D.C.: The World Bank, 2004a (http://lnweb18.worldbank.org/oed/oeddoclib. nsf/DocUNIDViewForJavaSearch/67433EC6C181C22385256E7F007 3BA1C/$file/influential_evaluations_ecd.pdf, accessed July 2005).

The World Bank, *Monitoring & Evaluation: Some Tools, Methods, and Approaches*, Washington, D.C.: The World Bank, 2004b (http:// lnweb18.worldbank.org/oed/oeddoclib.nsf/24cc3bb1f94ae11c85256808 006a0046/a5efbb5d776b67d285256b1e0079c9a3/$FILE/MandE_tools _methods_approaches.pdf, accessed July 2005).

____. *2003 Annual Review of Development Effectiveness: The Effectiveness of Bank Support for Policy Reform*, Washington, D.C.: The World Bank, 2004c (http://www.worldbank.org/oed/arde2003/; accessed July 2005).

____. *World Development Indicators 1998*, Washington, D.C.: The World Bank, 1998.

The World Bank Group, "Costs of Evaluation," October 4, 2004a (http://web.worldbank.org/WEBSITE/EXTERNAL/NEWS/0,,content MDK:20266739%7EmenuPK:34457%7EpagePK:34370%7EpiPK:344 24%7EtheSitePK:4607,00.html; accessed July 2005).

____. "Evaluation . . . A Necessary Science," 2004b (http://web. worldbank.org/WBSITE/EXTERNAL/NEWS/0,,contentMDK:202667

30~menuPK:34457~pagePK:34370~piPK:34424~theSitePK:4607,00.ht ml; accessed July 2005).

World Health Organization, "Report of a 'Lessons Learnt' Workshop on the Six ProTEST Pilot Projects in Malawi, South Africa and Zambia; February 3–6, 2003," Durban, South Africa: WHO, 2004.

____. "Progress Towards Global Immunization Goals—2001: Summary Presentation of Key Findings," PowerPoint presentation, 2003a.

____. *Progress Towards Immunization Goals,* Geneva, Switzerland: WHO, 2003b.

____. *An Expanded DOTS Framework for Effective Tuberculosis Control,* Geneva, Switzerland: WHO, 2002a.

____. State of the World's Vaccine and Immunization, Geneva, Switzerland: Department of Vaccines and Biologicals, WHO, WHO/V&B/02.21, 2002b.

____. *What is DOTS? A Guide to Understanding the WHO-Recommended TB Control Strategy Known as DOTS,* Geneva: WHO, 1999, pp. 1–33.

World Medical Association (WMA), *Declaration of Helsinki, Ethical Principles for Medical Research Involving Human Subjects,* adopted by the 18th WMA General Assembly, Helsinki, Finland, June 1964; amended by 29th WMA General Assembly, Tokyo, Japan, October 1975; 35th WMA General Assembly, Venice, Italy, October 1983; 41st WMA General Assembly, Hong Kong, September 1989; 48th WMA General Assembly, Somerset West, Republic of South Africa, October 1996; and 52nd WMA General Assembly, Edinburgh, Scotland, October 2000.

Wright, John, John Walley, Aby Philip, Suresh Pushpananthan, Elijah Dlamini, James Newell, and Sweetness Dlamini, "Direct Observation of Treatment for Tuberculosis: A Randomized Controlled Trial of Community Health Workers Versus Family Members," *Tropical Medicine & International Health,* Vol. 9, No. 5, May 2004, p. 559.

Yusuf, S., "Clinical Research and Trials in Developing Countries," *Statistics in Medicine,* Vol. 21, October 15, 2002, pp. 2859–2867.

Zwarenstein, M., J. H. Schoeman, C. Vundule, C. J. Lombard, and M. Tatley, "Randomised Controlled Trial of Self-Supervised and Directly Observed Treatment of Tuberculosis," *Lancet,* October 24, 1998, pp. 1340–1343.